boosting
your
digestive
health

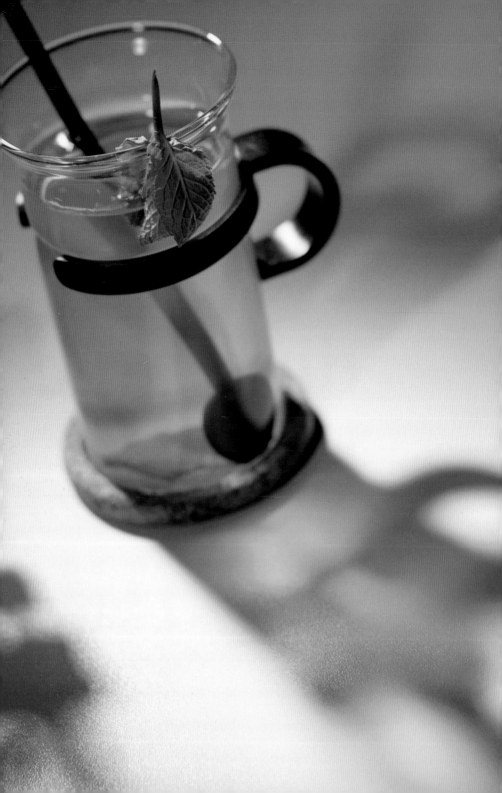

boosting your digestive health

Mark Kane

Dr. Len Saputo, Editor and Consultant

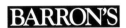

First edition for the United States and Canada published in 2002 by
Barron's Educational Series, Inc.

Publisher's note: Before following any advice or exercises contained in
this book, it is recommended that you consult your doctor if you suffer
from any health problems or special conditions. The publisher cannot
accept responsibility for any injuries or damage incurred as a result of
following the advice given in this book.

Additional titles in the *Options for Health* series:
Beating Sports Injuries
Beating the Years

All inquiries should be addressed to:
Barron's Educational Series, Inc.
250 Wireless Boulevard
Hauppauge, NY 11788
http://www.barronseduc.com

Library of Congress Catalog Card Number 2001096142

International Standard Book Number 0-7641-1903-6

Picture Credits
Front cover Corbis Stockmarket/Owen Franken; 2 Photodisc; 10 Photodisc; 19 ImageState;
26 Science Photo Library/BSIP, Laurent/Yakou; 32 Photodisc; 38 Photodisc; 44 Science
Photo Library/USDA; 50 Photodisc; 54 Science Photo Library/BSIP, Taulin; 58 Science
Photo Library/TH Foto-Werbung; 63 Photodisc; 67 Science Photo Library/Susan Leavines;
71 Robert Harding Picture Library/CNRI/Phototake NYC; 72 Photodisc; 80 Photodisc; 83
Photodisc; 84 Powerstock; 92 Photodisc; 95 Photodisc; 98 Photodisc; 101 Photodisc; 102
Octopus Publishing Group Ltd./Hamlyn/James Merrell; 105 Photodisc; 108 Corbis/Phil
Schermeister; 111 Photodisc; 114 Octopus Publishing Group Ltd./Hamlyn/C. Bowling;
119 Science Photo Library/Gusto Productions; 125 Photodisc; 127 Photodisc; 128
Photodisc; 137 Photodisc; 138 ImageState

Printed and bound by Toppan Printing Company, China
9 8 7 6 5 4 3 2 1

contents

foreword

If you have been searching for a complete resource that provides easy-to-understand information about what the digestive tract is, how it functions in health, common digestive illnesses, and what can be done to restore and maintain optimal digestive function, this book is for you. Mark Kane does this from the perspective of different health care disciplines with a view to treating the whole person—body, mind, and spirit.

Boosting Your Digestive Health takes a common-sense approach. It emphasizes the importance of self-care, recognizing that the medicine of the future begins with taking responsibility for your own health through lifestyle management: diet, exercise, stress reduction, and avoidance of toxic substances. Kane also presents an in-depth look at the most common digestive disorders, presenting integrative solutions when lifestyle alone is insufficient.

A well-functioning digestive tract is one of the most important factors that determines your health and vitality—it is impossible to be healthy unless your digestive tract is healthy. It has the responsibility of delivering the nutrition that all of your cells require to function properly. Think about it. If all of your cells are healthy, how can you be sick? You can only be as healthy as your cells!

Each of our cells is a microscopic industrial plant. Every day they require thousands of raw materials (found in the food we consume), in order to generate energy, and manufacture products that restore and maintain normal cell metabolism. In this day and age, where whole, natural, and unprocessed foods are not commonly consumed, proper nutrition is a challenge. Several large studies on thousands of normal people have consistently documented that widespread nutritional deficiencies exist in all modern civilizations.

There is a second way that cells can malfunction—when they are nourished with chemicals, microbes, or other toxic substances that can disrupt normal cell physiology. In this era of biochemical technology, we have polluted our food, water, and air with tens of thousands of chemicals that have never before been inside a human body, and to which we've simply not had time to adapt. Unless we pay more attention to sustaining a natural environment with clean food, water, and air, we will continue to poison ourselves on a daily basis.

You have all heard, "You are what you eat." While there is truth in this, it is only part of a larger story. You can eat the most nutritious food and add the most powerful supplements to your diet, but if your digestive tract is not digesting and absorbing properly, optimal nourishment cannot be delivered to the cells of your body. In actuality, you are what you eat, digest, absorb, deliver to the cells of your body, and, finally, what your cells then assimilate.

There is far more to digestive function than simply delivering nutrients to your cells. The intestinal tract is a major interface between the external world and your inner milieu, and what is presented to this surface includes more than food. There are thousands of toxic chemicals that find their way into the food and water that we consume. The intestinal tract has the awesome responsibility of keeping these toxins from entering the internal body, where they can upset cellular physiology and cause disease.

The intestinal tract harbors more than 500 different species of microbes, accounting for trillions of microorganisms that produce more metabolic activity than any organ system in the human body. These microbes live in a complex microecology that is extremely sensitive and has profound effects on its human host. When the delicate balance in this ecology is upset by antibiotics, certain drugs, or other toxic substances, digestion, absorption, immune function, liver detoxification, and other important metabolic functions may become seriously disrupted and result in digestive and other disorders.

Boosting Your Digestive Health includes simple but comprehensive descriptions of the main tests used in mainstream and alternative medicine that are used to evaluate symptoms and diagnose digestive disorders. This information will enable you to make informed decisions and work more intelligently with your health care practitioners.

Today's health care is becoming a collaborative process where dialogue between patients and physicians is expected. We are learning that the best way to ensure good health comes from taking more responsibility for making decisions about our health care needs. Mark Kane has provided a very useful resource for anyone with digestive problems, as well as for those interested in learning more about living a healthier life.

Dr. Len Saputo, Editor

introduction

Just about everyone has experienced the discomfort of disordered digestion. One of life's great pleasures—eating and drinking—can sometimes be taken to excess, and we pay the price with an upset digestive system the next day. For others, digestive problems are a daily burden, and millions of dollars are spent on over-the-counter and prescription medicines to try to control the symptoms. Complementary medicines have become increasingly popular, and many remedies that can be safely used to treat digestive problems are available. All these treatments have a place, but what many people need is a better understanding of why their digestive system gives them problems and what they can do to prevent, cure, or manage digestive disease. Just as important as any remedy or treatment is knowing how you can adjust your lifestyle, diet, and any other factors that can lead to digestive illness.

This book is designed to help you gain a better understanding of the causes of digestive problems. It explains how the symptoms are produced, why the symptoms are present, and what strategy you need to adopt to treat the causes.

The book starts with a journey through the digestive tract. Although digestion is a robust activity, it remains mostly hidden from us once we swallow our food—that is, unless we are experiencing problems. By understanding how a normal digestive system works, we can better understand what can go wrong. The next part of the book explains simply and clearly how symptoms occur and what causes them. Although many digestive conditions are relatively benign—that is, they are not a matter of life or death—some diseases have very serious consequences. The key symptoms that would alert you to this possibility are highlighted. The next section describes the conditions or diseases that underlie the symptoms. These conditions are what your doctor or other health professional will try to diagnose. The tests they will use for this diagnosis are explained.

The second part of the book, Options for Health, starts with broad guidelines about healthy living. There are suggestions for what you should eat and what you should avoid. How you eat is also important: Simple things like chewing your food properly and not eating on the run can do wonders for your digestive health. *Stress* is a recurrent word when it comes to health, and this part of the book explains how stress can affect the digestive system and what you can do to manage your stress more effectively. Exercise is an important ingredient in health, and broader issues—such as relationships, career, and life direction—also play a part. Although these topics are beyond the scope of this book, some ideas are introduced to help you evaluate whether these issues might be contributing to your digestive problems.

This book details a range of simple remedies, such as healthy foods, nutritional supplements, and herbal remedies. Some simple indications are provided for self-prescribing homeopathy, and the most important over-the-counter and prescription medicines are explained. In the final section, the basic principles of various therapies are explained as well as their recommended use. You will also get an idea of what to expect if you see a professional practitioner from these disciplines, which include acupuncture, homeopathy, naturopathy, and orthodox and integrated medicine.

However you choose to use this book, whether it is dipping in at random, following the links between chapters, or reading from cover to cover, you will find a wealth of ideas, explanations, and sound advice. May it bring you good health.

How the tabs work

Each section has been allocated its own color, found at the bottom right-hand corner of each right-hand page in that section page. Throughout the book, each right-hand page will also show solid tabs referring you to the sections where you will find more useful information. For example, here you are being referred to the chapter on Lifestyle Changes.

Symptoms

Conditions

Tests

Lifestyle changes

Simple remedies

Therapies

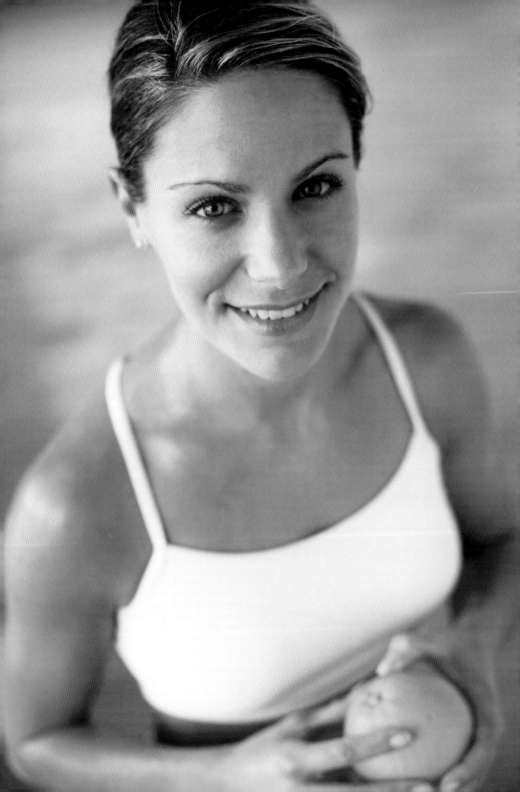

understanding
digestive
health

Our understanding of digestive health has advanced hugely over the last 20 years, enabling earlier diagnosis and better treatment of digestive conditions—and, in many cases, enabling individuals to treat themselves using a wide variety of techniques, therapies, and medicines. More than any other system in the human body, the digestive system lets us know when its organs are functioning well—hunger and a need to empty the bowels being two normal daily signals. But these organs also quickly let us know when something is not right. This section will give you a sound understanding of how your digestive system works, what can go wrong, and what your symptoms could mean.

the **digestive** system

There is much more to the digestive system than the stomach and bowels. Starting from the mouth this system extends through to the anus and includes various glands, organs, and even resident bacterial populations that work for the body. The system performs the vital role of digesting and assimilating nutrition as well as disposing of waste.

Many people have only a vague idea of what happens once food is swallowed, because from this point the digestive system functions without conscious control, and the nervous system takes over. The following section takes you on a tour through your digestive tract and outlines the process of normal digestion. This should help you to understand why digestive problems are so common and explain the basis for preventing and treating common problems.

The mind

Before food even passes the lips, the aroma and thought of food stimulates the digestive juices in the mouth and stomach to prepare the body for the intake of food. If you are anxious or distracted, then the mouth and stomach does not receive the signal to prepare for food. The mind prepares the body to accept and digest food, and if you eat in a relaxed and unhurried way, you digest your food more effectively.

The mouth

The food you take into your mouth is first chopped and ground into smaller pieces by the teeth. This chewing stimulates the salivary glands to release large quantities of enzyme-rich saliva, which mixes with the food. These enzymes start the chemical breakdown of food, particularly carbohydrates, which are sugary and starchy foods such as potatoes and fruit. If there is insufficient moisture in the food, it is likely to be difficult to swallow. The moisture in the saliva makes it easier to move the food around in the mouth and helps carry the small ball of chopped-up food down the esophagus to the stomach.

The esophagus

When you swallow, muscles in the mouth push the food through a ring of muscle at the back of the throat known as the esophageal sphincter. This one-way valve prevents food from being regurgitated back into the mouth. The esophagus connects the throat to the stomach and in an adult is about 10 in (25 cm) long. Once the food is inside the esophagus, a most extraordinary activity takes place. A wavelike motion takes place in the muscles as they relax in front of the food, allowing it to pass forward and contract behind the food to push it along. This pattern of movement is called peristalsis—a process that carries on right through the digestive tract. As the food reaches the lower end of the esophagus, the buildup of pressure activates another muscular one-way valve called the lower esophageal sphincter (LES). When you are not eating, this valve remains tightly sealed to prevent the contents of the stomach from being forced back into the esophagus and creating heartburn.

The stomach

Looking a bit like a large sausage, the stomach lies in the upper left corner of your abdomen under the ribs. This hollow muscular sac is about 10 in (25 cm) long and expands considerably when food enters. Well before food passes into the stomach, the stomach has already begun to secrete juices. Normally several quarts a day are produced.

The stomach has three main functions. First, it acts as a storage container for swallowed food. Second, the stomach churns and gyrates to promote the mixing of the food with the digestive secretions, including hydrochloric acid and pepsin. It is somewhat surprising that such vigorous churning is not usually felt. This is because the stomach has relatively few sensory nerve fibers compared to other parts of the body, such as the skin. The soupy liquid produced by the mixing of food particles with digestive juice is called chyme. This mixture remains in the stomach anywhere between 45 minutes and 4 hours before passing into the small intestine. Several factors influence the emptying of the stomach, including the nature of the food and the degree of muscular activity in the stomach and small intestine. If the hydrochloric acid secretions are insufficient, the digestion of proteins and the absorption of vitamin B_{12} are impaired. This in turn slows the movement of chyme into the small intestine. High-fat and high-fiber foods tend to slow the emptying time. The third function of the stomach is to destroy most of the bacteria and other microorganisms

THE DIGESTIVE APPARATUS

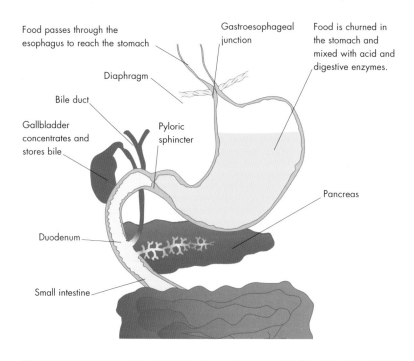

Food passes through the esophagus to reach the stomach

Gastroesophageal junction

Food is churned in the stomach and mixed with acid and digestive enzymes.

Diaphragm

Bile duct

Gallbladder concentrates and stores bile

Pyloric sphincter

Pancreas

Duodenum

Small intestine

Ingested food passes down the esophagus into the stomach, where it is churned and mixed with digestive juices secreted by the stomach lining. More digestive enzymes are added to the food in the duodenum.

that may have entered the body with the food. Hydrochloric acid is a powerful corrosive agent that kills most microorganisms it comes in contact with and activates the protein-digesting enzyme pepsin. The hydrochloric acid would dissolve the stomach itself were it not for a barrier of sticky, neutral mucus attached to the stomach wall. The stomach wall is highly impermeable, and most substances are absorbed into the blood when they reach the small intestine. The exceptions to this are water, electrolytes, alcohol, and certain drugs, such as aspirin. Eventually the liquidized food is pushed onward into the small intestine through another muscular valve, the pyloris.

The small intestine

The small intestine is the longest part of the digestive tract and is where the major digestive processes take place. It resembles a coiled-up garden hose and is 16–20 ft (5–6 m) long in an adult. It has three distinct parts. The duodenum lies just after your stomach and is about 12 in (30 cm) long. It is followed by the jejunum and the ileum, which connects to the large intestine. When food enters the duodenum, it is still highly acid from the stomach juices. To prevent the acid from burning the sensitive tissues, the pancreas secretes digestive juices rich in bicarbonates into the duodenum.

It takes 2–5 hours for the chyme to pass all the way through the small intestine. If all the many tiny folds called villi were flattened out, the surface area would cover a tennis court. It is over this surface area that nutrients are absorbed into the bloodstream. The villi produce enzymes to help absorb nutrients that pass through the villi into the body. If the small intestine is not functioning properly, it can lead to multiple nutritional deficiencies. This happens in conditions such as celiac disease. The villi also perform an important function of blocking the absorption of substances that the body does not require, such as chemicals, bacterial products, and large food molecules that have not been completely broken down. Certain foods and medications such as anti-inflammatory drugs make the villi more permeable to unwanted molecules. The body then responds to these foreign substances and mounts an immune response. This immune response is linked to conditions such as food sensitivities, arthritis, skin problems, migraine headaches, and chronic fatigue syndrome.

Gut-associated lymphatic tissue

There is a great potential for foreign substances to enter the bloodstream through the digestive tract, which is why much of the body's immune system is located in or around the gut. Secretory IgA (Ig means immunoglobulin, and A describes the class of antibody), which is present in the mucosa of the gastrointestinal lining, acts as first stage in immune defense by identifying and binding foreign substances. When foreign substances come in contact with the intestinal lining, specialized immune system cells called Peyer's patches screen the molecules, and if they are identified as harmful, the immune response is activated, and B cells and T cells (immune cells) are released to destroy the foreign "antigen." If the immune system is depressed—due to stress, infection, or a deficiency of a nutrient such as vitamin A, then foreign substances may breach these primary defenses. The result of this is that the immune system seeks out the molecules entering the bloodstream and locks them up in immune complexes that may be deposited in different body tissues, such as joints. This is the connection between the digestive system and arthritis.

The pancreas

Your pancreas has two main functions. The first is to secrete digestive juices into the duodenum; the second, to release insulin and glucagon directly into the bloodstream, where they help regulate the metabolism and blood sugar levels. The alkaline bicarbonate, which the pancreas secretes into the duodenum, neutralizes the highly acidic food passing from the stomach and prevents the acid from burning the sensitive duodenal lining. The pancreas also manufactures and secretes specific enzymes to digest fats, carbohydrates, and proteins. Lipase breaks down fats into fatty acids and glycerol. Amylase splits carbohydrates into simple sugars, and protease breaks the links between the amino acids that make up protein. When the food has been broken down into these components, they can be absorbed into the bloodstream. Without sufficient enzymes, you can not digest your food efficiently. Low secretion of pancreatic enzymes can lead to deficiencies of specific nutrients such as vitamin B_{12}.

The pancreas also controls blood sugar levels through the release of the hormones glucagon and insulin. Glucagon raises low blood sugar levels, and insulin decreases high blood sugar levels. Taking carbohydrates causes a rise in blood sugar levels. If the carbohydrates are slow-burning ones, the increase in blood sugar levels is gradual. The pancreas then releases insulin, and the sugar moves out of the blood into the tissues. If the release of insulin is impaired, a condition known as type 1 diabetes mellitus develops where the blood sugar level remains too high.

The liver and gallbladder

The liver and gallbladder also pour their secretions into the duodenum. The liver is an extraordinary organ that performs more than 500 functions. This chemical factory and detoxification plant sits under the lower ribs on the right side of the body and weighs about 4.4 lb (2 kg). It has many roles, including filtering and processing chemicals in food, storing nutrients, and breaking down old blood cells and hormones that the body no longer requires. Through a complex series of enzyme reactions, the liver makes nutrients more accessible.

Especially important for the digestion is the manufacture of bile. This greenish yellow liquid is made up of bile salts, cholesterol, and lecithin. Bile is secreted along the biliary tree into the duodenum to help the digestion of fats and fat-soluble vitamins. It does this by breaking down large globules into smaller ones, which provide more surface area for the fat-digesting enzymes to work on. Bile also helps transport wastes from the blood and promotes the incorporation of water into the stool. Without sufficient bile, the stool can become hard and difficult to pass.

The gallbladder is a small sac, about 2 in (6 cm) long, lying next to the liver. The biliary tree connects it to the liver and the duodenum. The liver secretes about 2 pints (1 liter) of bile into the biliary tree each day. When the body is not digesting food, the bile produced passes into the gallbladder, which concentrates the bile by removing water. When foods that contain fats enter the duodenum, a hormone signals the gallbladder to contract and release the concentrated bile into the duodenum.

With the combined juices of the liver, gallbladder, and pancreas, as well as the secretions from the wall of the small intestine, the digestive activity is intense. To bring the food particles in maximum contact with the surfaces of the small intestine, the muscular wave passing though the digestive tract carries the chyme through the duodenum in small clusters to the jejunum, where digestion is largely completed. The final section of the small intestine is called the ileum, where the remaining nutrients from the food are absorbed. The waste matter then passes through another muscular ring called the ileocecal valve into the large intestine. The passage of food through the small intestine takes anywhere from $1/2$–3 hours, depending on the food consumed.

The large intestine

Also known as the colon, the large intestine is 3–6 ft (1–2 m) long. The large intestine stores then removes waste that your body is unable to digest. By the time food residue reaches the large intestine, your body has absorbed most of the nutrients it can. What remains is water, electrolytes such as sodium and chloride, indigestible plant fiber, the dead cells shed from the lining of the digestive tract, and a massive bacterial population. These trillions of helpful bacteria are called probiotics and weigh up to 2.2 lb (1 kg). Probiotic bacteria are sometimes described as a body organ because they produce several vital functions for the body. They lower the pH of the large intestine, making the environment unfavorable for disease-producing microbes. Their activity encourages the peristaltic wavelike motion through the bowel. They also affect the digestion of vitamins A, B, and K as well as lactic acid in milk. Probiotic bacteria ferment the indigestible dietary fiber. This fermentation produces butyric acid, the main energy source for the cells of the colon. Low butyric acid levels have been associated with inflammatory bowel disease and colon cancer.

During the 12–24 hours when food waste passes through the large intestine, most of the water from the waste is absorbed, typically more than 2 pt (1 liter) a day. If the chyme passes through the large intestine too quickly, water will not be absorbed, resulting in diarrhea. If the forming stool remains too long in the large intestine, it will become dry and hard, leading to constipation. The normal stool is made up of two-thirds water, undigested fiber, and food products; the other third is made up of living and dead bacteria. Some of these bacteria cause food products to ferment and produce gas. When sulfur-rich foods, such as garlic and cabbage, are consumed, the gas has an unpleasant odor.

The anus

At the end of the digestive system, the stool is passed through the final muscular sphincter, which is the anus. The coordination of relaxation of the anal sphincter and pressure against the rectal walls by the stool, which, if necessary can be accentuated by contraction of the abdominal muscles, leads to the passing of the stool. If the tissues here are strained by constipation, hemorrhoids, bleeding, and pain may develop.

What can go wrong

The ordinary digestive system is pretty robust and will tolerate indiscretions and excesses without much complaint, but there is a limit. Lifestyle and poor nutritional habits weaken the digestive system and cause many of the digestive problems that afflict more than a third of the population.

When people live rushed and busy lifestyles, it is too easy to allow insufficient time for eating and digesting. Eating on the run or gulping food without proper chewing neither prepares the food for the body or the body for the food and may lead to indigestion or poor absorption of nutrients. When an individual is under a high level of stress, the body goes into alarm mode, and blood is directed away

Living a hectic modern lifestyle, eating on the run, and enduring high levels of stress can all trigger attacks of indigestion.

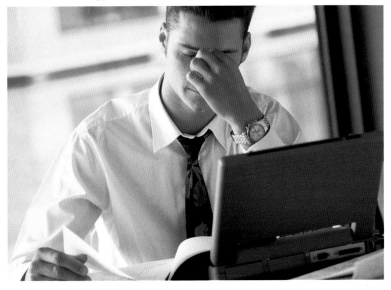

from the digestive organs to the muscles as the body prepares for fight or flight. This state of alarm is not conducive to the production of digestive enzymes or the proper functioning of the peristaltic wave that passes through the tract. Signs and symptoms like indigestion and bloating, abdominal cramps, diarrhea, and constipation may be the consequence of living with high levels of stress.

This is not to suggest that the cure for all digestive problems lies in the mind. What goes into the body in the form of food has a powerful influence on digestive function. Over the last century, the western diet has changed dramatically. The typical Western diet is high in saturated fats and low in fiber. Insufficient levels of fiber slow down the transit time of food through the gut, which can lead to constipation. This problem is compounded when salt intake is excessive and insufficient fluids are taken.

The profile of fatty foods consumed in the Western diet is far from ideal. High intake of fats, particularly saturated fats, is a primary factor in gallbladder and heart disease. The body does need fats. As well as being a concentrated source of energy, they provide building blocks for the body to make other chemicals and hormones. They are also needed for the transport, breakdown, and excretion of cholesterol.

Part of the problem is the kinds of fats that are consumed. Over the last 2 decades, there has been a mass campaign of health promotion to reduce intake of fats, which has been reinforced by the marketing of fat-free and low-fat food products. In spite of this, the incidence of obesity has increased dramatically over the last decade, and more than one of every five people are now classified as obese. This means that they are 30 percent or more above their ideal weight. This is partly a dietary problem because too many calories in the form of sugars and fats are being consumed.

Insufficient exercise is also a problem. As well as burning calories and stimulating metabolism, exercise aids digestion. Exercise also relieves stress, and because it encourages deep breathing, the digestive organs are massaged, helping to maintain their proper peristaltic rhythm. The effect of excessive body weight on the digestive organs drags down the organs and alters the passage of food and secretions in the gut. If the organs lose their natural rhythmicity due to mechanical strain, blood flow through the area is decreased.

Although there is reasonably good evidence to suggest that a modest alcohol intake has some health-protective properties, consumption of alcohol in excessive quantities undoubtedly undermines health and damages the organs of digestion, especially the stomach, liver, and pancreas. Alcohol can irritate the stomach lining and relax the sphincter that prevents acid rising up from the stomach into the esophagus. When acid reaches the esophagus, it burns the sensitive tissues and leads to what is commonly called heartburn.

Smoking is another well-known cause of digestive problems. Smokers have a much greater likelihood of suffering from heartburn. This is because nicotine in tobacco increases stomach acid production and decreases sodium bicarbonate production, which neutralizes the stomach acid when it reaches the duodenum. It also relaxes the sphincters, making it easier for the acid to pass up into the esophagus and burn the tissues.

Many medications have an adverse effect on digestion. Over-the-counter drugs, such as aspirin and ibuprofen (nurofen), and prescription nonsteroidal anti-inflammatory drugs (NSAIDs) can damage the lining of the stomach and cause bleeding. Stomach pain, nausea, stomach bleeding, and ulcers can result from using these drugs regularly or from exceeding the recommended dosage. Strong opiate analgesics can be very constipating. Other prescription drugs like antihypertensives for high blood pressure can lead to diarrhea or constipation. Antibiotics kill beneficial bacteria as well as harmful bacteria, which disturbs the ecology of the gut. In the short-term, such disturbance may result in diarrhea or constipation. In the long-term, it can contribute to conditions as diverse as fibromyalgia and food intolerance.

When medications are used more than occasionally to treat minor digestive disturbances, the adverse effects of the medication can lead to further problems and further intake of medications. Breaking this vicious cycle typically requires a re-evaluation of lifestyle, diet, and stress levels. When symptoms persist, it is important to seek a professional opinion. The symptoms of digestive distress rarely indicate a serious illness, such as stomach or bowel cancer. A qualified health professional, such as a family doctor or naturopath, will be able to recognize if your symptoms suggest a serious illness and require further investigation.

signs and symptoms

All of us have experienced disordered digestion at some time in our lives, and over half the population suffers from some form of indigestion more than once a month. Although many symptoms pass fairly quickly and do not indicate an underlying illness, it is important to recognize when to seek professional advice. This section describes the signs and symptoms of digestive disorder, and outlines the possible underlying causes.

Difficulty swallowing

Most of us swallow our food without a second thought, but difficulty swallowing can be a distressing symptom that can afflict some individuals every time they have a meal. The sense that food is sticking in the throat or chest is known as dysphagia. An occasional episode is generally not serious and can result from insufficient chewing, hurried eating, or stress.

A persistent difficulty swallowing requires a professional evaluation. The source of the problem may be in one of two areas—either the pharynx or the esophagus. Pharyngeal dysphagia is usually the result of a stroke or neurological disorder such as Parkinson's disease.

Esophageal dysphagia is more common and the sensation is like having food stuck in the esophagus, with a sense of pressure or pain in the chest. This is likely to be accompanied by painful swallowing and, perhaps, a sore throat and persistent cough. The causes are of two kinds. The first is narrowing of the passageway through which food passes and the second decreased motility and weakness of the muscles that propel the food down into the stomach. If stomach acid reaches the esophagus, its sensitive tissues are irritated. Over time, this can lead to scarring of the lower esophagus. The passage may become narrowed and have difficulty stretching to accommodate food. Other causes of obstructive dysphagia are tumors, burns from radiation treatment, and the formation of a band of tissues in the lower esophagus called Schatzki's ring. Motility disorders include sclerodema and achalasia.

Treatment Various treatments are available, but the choice depends upon the cause.

If the dysphagia is a result of a stroke or a neurological condition such as Parkinson's disease, then working with a speech and language therapist or physical therapist specializing in this area can help the individual to develop techniques for more effective swallowing.

Some physical therapists have developed specialized techniques to stretch the tissues surrounding the esophagus and re-educate the muscles to more effectively coordinate the propelling of food into the stomach. Another treatment used by gastroenterologists is the insertion of a long, flexible tube called an endoscope down into the esophagus. An inflatable balloon is passed through the endoscope, and the balloon is inflated to stretch the narrowed tissues.

If the dysphagia is a result of acid reflux, then medication or herbal treatment to reduce stomach-acid output may help. If spasm of the esophageal muscles is a problem, then muscle relaxants may help.

Diet Foods that are dry and chunky tend to aggravate dysphagia. It is important to chew food thoroughly to break it down and mix it with the saliva. Soft foods such as soups or puréed dishes are easier to swallow. Small rather than large meals create less difficulty.

Chest pain and heartburn

People develop chest pain for various reasons, and those experiencing it for the first time often worry that the problem is due to the heart. Although recognizing a heart problem is important, many structures in the chest can produce pain and discomfort, and heart disease is not on the top of the list of possible diagnoses. Other organs and tissues that can cause chest pain include the lungs, pleura, chest wall, esophagus, stomach, gallbladder, spine, ribs, and muscles. Emotional pain may be experienced in the chest, in the absence of disease or detectable dysfunction of the body. Hyperventilation and upper-chest breathing can also lead to chest pain.

Heartburn is used to describe a burning sensation in the center of the chest. It may start in the upper abdomen and radiate to the throat. A sour taste can occur in the mouth from acid regurgitation. Acid is normally prevented from backing up to the esophagus by the esophageal sphincter. This ring of muscle acts as a valve, which only opens when you swallow. Stomach acid that reaches the esophagus can burn and corrode the sensitive tissues. This produces the sensation known as heartburn. For some people, the symptom may be minor, but for others, it may be severe and lead to scarring of the esophageal tissues.

There are many reasons why heartburn occurs, such as being overweight, overeating, or lying down after eating. All of these things create an upward pressure of the stomach against the esophageal sphincter that may trigger it to open. Certain foods may trigger an attack in sensitive individuals. Alcohol, caffeine, and tobacco relax the esophageal sphincter, making it easier for acid to reach the esophagus. Having a hiatal hernia has long been considered a predisposing cause of heartburn, although opinions are now changing on this. A hiatal hernia occurs when the top portion of the stomach pushes up through the opening in the diaphragm so that part of the stomach is in the chest. A small hiatal hernia is unlikely to cause problems (in fact, this common condition causes no symptoms), but a large hernia may displace the esophageal sphincter from its position against the diaphragm. If the pressure keeping the sphincter closed is reduced, then acid will more easily pass into the esophagus. The hernia then becomes a reservoir for gastric acid, which can easily splash up into the esophagus as you move about or lean forward.

Occasional bouts of heartburn are common and are usually caused by overeating or drinking too much alcohol. However, heartburn can also stem from a more serious condition, such as gastroesophageal reflux disease (GERD) or a heart problem. If the heartburn is occasional and related to overeating or drinking too much alcohol, then treating yourself with lifestyle changes or over-the-counter medications or herbal remedies is quite safe. If the heartburn is persistent and there is referred pain into the arm, see your medical practitioner without delay. Esophageal spasm produces intense chest pain that can seem identical to cardiac pain, so a thorough cardiac evaluation may be required to differentiate the cause of the pain. It may be, however, that the heartburn is a warning of angina or a heart attack.

To find out more about GERD, see Conditions section, p.36. For gallstones, see Conditions section, p.59.

Bloating and flatulence

Three factors control the amount of gas within the digestive system: swallowing of air, the foods eaten, and the microorganisms within the gut.

Bloating is the buildup of gas in the stomach and intestines and may also be accompanied by abdominal pain. Air and gas tend to accumulate as a normal part of digestion. It is usual to swallow some air when you eat food, but the amount increases if you eat too quickly or talk while you eat. For some people, swallowing air becomes a nervous habit, even when they are not eating or drinking. Depending on whether the air goes up or down, the outcome is belching or flatulence, which is a normal response and the body's way of expelling excess air. Bloating may also result from eating a lot of fatty foods, because these slow down the emptying of the stomach, increase the sensation of fullness, and allow foods more time to ferment and produce excessive gas.

Certain foods and drinks, such as beer and carbonated drinks, tend to promote the formation of gas within the digestive tract. Gas also occurs when the intestines are unable to break down the foods eaten. Intestinal bacteria begin to ferment the indigestible fiber in some foods, and gas is produced. This is normal and the health benefits of eating fiber-rich foods certainly compensate for a certain amount of gas. Often when a person introduces a fiber-rich diet, it can take a few weeks before the body adapts and produces less gas. The formation of excessive gas is only half of the problem. Fermentation of sulfur compounds in foods produces foul-smelling gas. Eggs, meat, beans, and onions are rich in sulfur compounds. Certain foods such as Jerusalem artichokes contain an insoluble starch called inulin, which cannot be digested and commonly causes uncomfortable flatulence.

The wrong balance of microorganisms in the gut can cause excessive and foul gases to be produced. If the passage of digested food through the bowel is sluggish and slow, the degree of fermentation increases, with an excess of gas being produced. The balance of microflora can be drastically disturbed by repeated courses of antibiotics and may require supplementation with beneficial acidophilus bacteria. The avoidance of constipation is an important part of correcting bloating and flatulence.

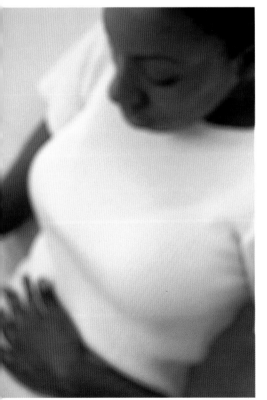

See the Conditions section for dysbiosis (p.46), irritable bowel syndrome (p.52), and gallbladder disease (p.59).

Indigestion

Indigestion is an ambiguous term that can mean different things to different people. It commonly refers to discomfort in the central upper abdomen related to the intake of food. The term is also used to describe a number of other signs and symptoms such as pain in the chest (heartburn), bloating, belching, and nausea.

Symptoms of indigestion are commonly felt in the upper abdomen.

Indigestion is a common symptom. The most common causes are eating and drinking to excess and excessive stress. If the cause is due to dietary indiscretions, then the occasional bout can be safely treated by making lifestyle changes or using over-the-counter medications or herbs.

Inflammation of the stomach (gastritis) may be responsible for the symptoms of indigestion. In fact, one of the most important causes of gastritis is the use of alcohol and medications such as aspirin and other anti-inflammatory drugs. The problem is made worse when the drugs are taken on an empty stomach, which eventually leads to ulceration of the stomach.

Persistent or severe indigestion may indicate a serious underlying problem, such as peptic ulcers. If the symptoms are severe or last for more than a couple of weeks, or if you experience the symptoms for the first time after age 40, then it is important to seek medical advice.

Less-common causes of indigestion include infection from spoiled food or unfamiliar bugs, which can lead to gastroenteritis, or inflammation of the lining of the stomach and intestines. However, the stomach is not the only organ responsible for the symptoms of indigestion. Gallbladder inflammation or pancreatic disease can disturb the digestive processes and lead to symptoms. See the Conditions section for gastroesophageal reflux disease (GERD) (p.36), ulcers (p.39), gallbladder disease (p.59). Also refer to the section about Lifestyle Changes (p.74).

Nausea and vomiting

A common cause of nausea and vomiting is viral or bacterial infection from spoiled food. The infection leads to inflammation of the lining of the stomach and intestines. Most people at some time eat or drink something that makes them feel nauseous. High levels of alcohol, drugs, or other toxins and the increased hormone levels that occur early in pregnancy can all trigger the symptoms.

Almost anything can make people feel nauseous or "sick to the stomach"— migraine headaches, emotional or physical trauma, or even an overdose of sun. Nausea and vomiting generally are not indications of serious disease, unless they persist or are accompanied by pain. However, there are more serious causes of nausea and vomiting such as meningitis and inner-ear disturbances.

To manage simple nausea and vomiting, avoid eating and drinking for a short time until the stomach has settled. It is essential that you avoid becoming dehydrated, so as you start to feel better, begin taking sips of water or suck ice chips. Weak tea or a herb tea, such as peppermint or chamomile tea, can help. When you do start eating again, choose simple foods that are easily digested (such as dry toast, rice, and fruits) rather than spicy or fatty foods. Avoid consuming anything that will irritate the gut, such as aspirin or anti-inflammatory drugs, alcohol, or caffeine.

For more information, consult the following in the Conditions section: ulcers and stomach pain (p.39) and gallbladder and liver disease (p.59). For treatments, see the Simple Remedies section, in particular, herbal medicine (p.112) and Homeopathy (p.116). Also see acupuncture and acupressure (p.124) in the Therapies section.

Abdominal pain

Most cases of abdominal pain stem from minor digestive upsets; however, if pain is severe and persistent, you should seek medical attention without delay. There are several causes of severe abdominal pain, and an expert diagnosis is required.

Consult a doctor if extreme pain persists for more than 4 hours or if you develop other symptoms. Occasional episodes of discomfort or moderate pain may occur from eating too much or from eating foods that are too fatty or that produce gas. Modifying the diet should be sufficient to prevent such episodes.

If the abdominal pain is accompanied by diarrhea, a likely cause is gastroenteritis. This inflammation of the digestive tract is caused by infection or food poisoning. The advice is similar to that given for treating nausea and vomiting caused by eating spoiled food: Avoid becoming dehydrated by maintaining adequate fluid intake. If you cannot drink large amounts of fluids, try taking

SEEK MEDICAL ADVICE

Pain experienced in the following areas may point to problems elsewhere in the body. You should consult your doctor for a full diagnosis.

- Navel area: appendix, small intestine
- Above the navel: stomach, small intestine, gallbladder, pancreas,
- Below navel: colon or, more commonly in women, urinary tract infection or pelvic inflammatory disease
- Right upper quadrant of the abdomen: gallbladder or pancreas
- Left lower quadrant: descending colon (diverticulitis or colitis)
- Right lower quadrant: colitis or, more seriously, appendicitis

SEEK MEDICAL ADVICE

!

Consult your doctor without delay if any of the following can be used to characterize your abdominal pain.

- *Severe or unexplained*
- *Getting worse*
- *Accompanied by fever, bleeding, or vomiting*
- *Recurrent or persistent*

frequent sips of water or tea. Peppermint tea and chamomile tea are helpful for simple digestive upsets. Slippery elm bark powder is soothing to the gut and helps heal the inflamed gut lining. When you do start eating, try simple foods, such as soups or rice. A viral or bacterial infection may last 1–2 days. If the symptoms persist or are accompanied by other symptoms, this may indicate a more serious condition.

The location of abdominal pain is at best a rough guide, and where the pain is felt may be quite remote from the source of the pain. This phenomenon known as reflex or referred pain makes diagnosis of abdominal pain challenging even for experts, and if the source of the pain is not clear from the history or examination, more tests may be required.

Diarrhea

Diarrhea is an increase in the fluidity or frequency of bowel movements and may be accompanied by cramping abdominal pain, bloating, nausea, or an urgent need to evacuate the bowels. The stools have passed through the small intestine and colon too quickly, or the gut lining is unable to absorb the excess fluids to make the stool firm. The causes include viral, bacterial, and parasitic infections; food intolerance; reactions to medicine; and intestinal diseases and disorders, such as irritable bowel syndrome. The occasional attack of diarrhea caused by a bacterial or viral infection normally settles within 1–3 days and does not require prescription medication. If the condition persists over a longer period, you should see your health professional. Diarrhea can cause dehydration, which means the body lacks enough fluid to function properly. Drink at least 2 pt (1 liter) of clear fluids daily to ensure that you do not become dehydrated. Appropriate fluids include water, weak tea, herbal infusions and drinks containing electrolytes such as rice and barley water, fresh vegetable juices (especially carrot and celery), miso broth, and other clear broths. Rice and barley water are made using 1 cup of grain to 2 pt (1 liter) of boiling water. Leave to steep for 20 minutes, then strain and drink throughout the day. Refrain from eating solid foods for a day, then gradually reintroduce easily digestible food (such as bananas, plain rice, boiled potatoes, toast, or crackers) before returning to your regular diet. Foods that are very spicy or fatty and beverages that contain caffeine or alcohol may prolong diarrhea and should be avoided until you have fully recovered. Some people are unable to digest certain components in foods, such as lactose, which is the sugar found in dairy products. This will lead to diarrhea.

Such medications as antibiotics, blood pressure medications, and antacids that contain magnesium can cause diarrhea. Diarrhea is sometimes a reaction to stress and when recurrent may be part of the irritable bowel syndrome.

In the Conditions section, see food allergies and intolerance (p.49), irritable bowel syndrome (p.52), celiac disease (p.55), and inflammatory bowel disease (p.56).

Constipation

Constipation is difficulty in emptying the bowels, due to the passage of small amounts of hard, dry bowel movements, every day or, more usually, fewer than three times a week. People who are constipated may find it painful to have a bowel movement. Other symptoms of constipation include feeling bloated, uncomfortable, and sluggish. Most people experience constipation occasionally, but for some people the symptoms are present most or all of the time. Constipation occurs when the colon absorbs too much water, leaving little for the stools to absorb, which then become hard and dry. This happens if the colon's muscle contractions are slow or sluggish, causing the stool to move through the colon too slowly.

Common causes of constipation The most common cause of constipation is a diet low in fiber. Foods high in fiber include vegetables and fruits, rice, and bread and pasta made with unrefined cereals.

It is important to have sufficient fluid intake. This adds bulk to stools, making bowel movements softer and easier to pass. Fiber acts as a sponge by absorbing water into the stool. People who have problems with constipation should ensure they drink at least 4 pt (2 liters) of clear fluids a day. The best sources are water, juice, and clear liquid broths. Beverages that contain caffeine (such as tea, coffee, and cola) or alcohol tend to have a diuretic effect, causing the fluid to pass through the urine.

Such medications as strong analgesics, antacids that contain aluminium, antidepressants, anticonvulsants, ferrous sulfate iron supplements, and diuretics can all be constipating.

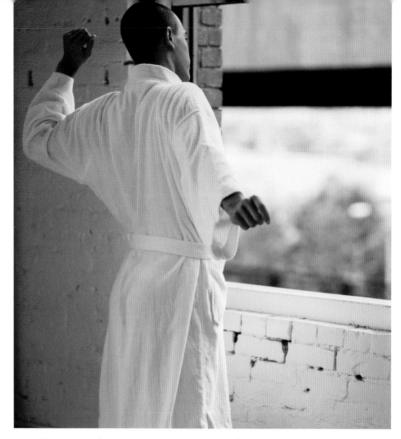

Your lifestyle can have a real impact on your digestive health.

Changes in lifestyle and routines Lack of exercise reduces the stimulation to the bowel and promotes constipation. It is well recognized that those who are bedridden tend to suffer more from constipation. Metabolism tends to slow with aging, and this results in reduced intestinal activity and muscle tone. Women may be constipated during pregnancy due to hormonal changes and the weight of the uterus pressing down on the bowel. Constipation may be a sign of hypothyroidism or magnesium deficiency. Traveling may also play a part because normal diet and routines are disrupted.

Ignoring the urge to have a bowel movement is a significant cause of constipation. Whether due to emotional stress, preoccupation with other things, or not wanting to use facilities outside the home, ignoring these urges can become habitual, and eventually the urges may no longer be felt. Some people then begin to rely on laxatives. When these drugs are used regularly, the bowel becomes lazy and increasingly reliant upon them for stimulation to action. By paying more attention to dietary and lifestyle factors, simple constipation—even if it is long-term—can be reversed, but specific conditions such as irritable bowel syndrome may be the cause. If the condition has existed for a long time, or if constipation is a recent change in your bowel habit, seek the opinion of your health care professional.

Refer to the whole section on Lifestyle Changes, beginning on p.74, and also make food your medicine (p.100) in the Simple Remedies section. Also see the section on irritable bowel syndrome (p.52) in the Conditions section.

Bleeding

Bleeding can become visible at both ends of the digestive tract. The causes may be minor, such as blood in the mouth from bleeding gums or small amounts of blood around the anus from bleeding hemorrhoids. However, bleeding in the digestive tract can also result from serious causes, such as peptic ulcers, damage to the intestinal lining, or even cancer. It is therefore important to seek the advice of your health care professional.

Blood from the mouth A small amount of bright red blood is likely to come from the gums rather than the stomach, but sometimes a tear in the lining of the esophagus can lead to fresh blood in the saliva or vomit. If the blood has been in the stomach for only a short time, it may be bright red. If the blood has been partially digested in the stomach, it will be dark brown or black and resemble coffee grounds.

Rectal bleeding Hemorrhoids are veins in the anus that are swollen with blood. They are the most common cause of lower-digestive tract bleeding. An increase of pressure from straining at stool may lead to bleeding, and bright red blood may be apparent after a bowel movement. Diverticular disease is a common cause of rectal bleeding. More serious causes of rectal bleeding are ulcerative colitis, Crohn's disease, and cancer. When the source of bleeding is farther up the digestive tract, more blood is mixed in with the stool, and it tends to be darker in color. Stools that are very dark or black may indicate bleeding from the upper digestive tract.

Various creams and suppositories that act locally to relieve inflammation and irritation are available. Rectal bleeding is aggravated by constipation and straining to pass stool, which is why it is important to ensure adequate fiber and fluids in the diet. The main risk with self-treatment of hemorrhoids is the delay in diagnosis of bowel cancer. Although bowel cancer is nowhere near as common as hemorrhoids, a delay in diagnosis and treatment could have serious consequences.

See irritable bowel syndrome (p.52) and inflammatory bowel disease (p.56) in the Conditions section.

Changes in weight

It is normal for body weight to fluctuate a little, even on a daily basis as you accumulate and shed fluids. In most cases, the reason people lose weight is that their calorie intake has changed, the level of their energy expenditure has increased, or their metabolic rate has increased. If, however, unintentionally you begin to lose more than 5 percent of your total body weight in a month or 10 percent in 6 months and you are not sure why this is happening, you should see your health care professional. If your diet contains enough calories but you are still losing weight, then you may not be absorbing your nutrients efficiently. The enzymes secreted from the mouth, stomach, and pancreas are crucial in breaking down fats, carbohydrates, and proteins. If the pancreas is not functioning effectively, then you will not have the enzymes to break down fats, carbohydrates, or proteins. Absorption follows after the breakdown of food, so if there are problems with the small intestine, then you may lose weight. Diseases affecting the small intestine include celiac disease (an intolerance to the gluten in wheat) and Crohn's disease (inflammatory bowel disease).

Diseases of the liver or cancers may also result in unintentional weight loss. If the thyroid is overactive, then an excess of the thyroid hormone thyroxine will circulate in the blood. This hormone speeds up the metabolic rate and causes you to burn more energy than you normally would. If, however, the thyroid is underactive, then you will tend to gain weight as your metabolic rate decreases. Overactivity of the thyroid is less common than underactivity, but it can occur. All of the above causes can be investigated, and appropriate tests need to be done to establish the precise causes.

See the Conditions section for inflammatory bowel disease (p.56), celiac disease (p.55), gallbladder and liver disease (p.59), and cancers of the digestive system (p.60).

When to seek professional advice

Most minor digestive disturbances can be self-treated by adjusting diet, lifestyle, or the occasional use of over-the-counter remedies, but it is important to recognize when you should seek professional help. If there is no improvement in your symptoms after such self-treatment, you should not delay getting a professional opinion. If you develop indigestion for the first time after age 40 or the indigestion is different from what you have experienced before, you may need evaluation and testing to rule out serious diseases like peptic ulcers and cancer. You should also seek advice if you notice any marked changes in your bowel habits.

If your symptoms are minor or if the cause is clearly overindulgence, seeking professional help may be unnecessary. If on the other hand the symptoms are severe or you do not understand what has caused them, then you should seek advice.

There are certain "red flag" symptoms that should alert you to the possibility of serious disease. Although these symptoms alone do not indicate serious disease, they should always be thoroughly checked out by a health care professional who is fully trained in medical diagnosis, such as your doctor or naturopath.

SEEK MEDICAL ADVICE FOR THESE SYMPTOMS

- *Unintentional weight loss*
- *Difficulty swallowing*
- *Vomit that contains blood or material that looks like coffee grounds*
- *Blood in your stools (the stools may look tarry)*
- *Indigestion while you are taking anti-inflammatory drugs*
- *Change in bowel habit*

conditions

The signs and symptoms described in the previous chapter may indicate any of a number of medical conditions. If symptoms persist, it is crucial that you seek medical advice for an accurate diagnosis and treatment. This chapter looks at the most common conditions, highlighting what can cause them and how they may be diagnosed and treated.

Gastroesophageal reflux disease

Gastroesophageal reflux disease (GERD) is the most common cause of indigestion. Although most people have experienced heartburn at some time, frequent heartburn can be a serious problem. GERD is a digestive disorder that affects the lower esophageal sphincter (LES), the muscle connecting the esophagus to the stomach. Many people, including pregnant women, suffer from heartburn or acid indigestion caused by GERD. The most common symptom is a burning sensation in the chest, going up to the throat.

When you swallow food, it travels down the esophagus, and the pressure of the food against the closed lower esophageal sphincter normally causes a relaxation of the sphincter, which allows the food to enter the stomach. The sphincter should remain closed at all other times to prevent stomach acid from reaching the sensitive tissues of the esophagus. If the stomach acid is allowed to travel back up to the esophagus, the symptoms of heartburn are produced.

The two main causes of this heartburn are an overrelaxed sphincter and a stomach that protrudes through the diaphragm, also known as a hiatal hernia. It is not always clear why some people have an overrelaxed sphincter, but several factors can play a part. Being overweight, drinking heavily, smoking, eating fatty, spicy, or acidic foods, and taking certain medications (such as drugs for asthma) can all relax the sphincter. If the stomach is full, and emptying into the duodenum is delayed, then acid may back up into the esophagus.

For some people, the symptoms are mild with only occasional upsets, whereas for others, the symptoms are severe, and the chest pain may cause concern about their hearts. If you have heartburn twice a week or more for several weeks or your usual symptoms are getting worse, you should see your health care professional. If you have heartburn with no other complications, you may be given lifestyle recommendations and treatment without further evaluation. If your symptoms are severe or there are additional symptoms, further evaluation may be required.

Establishing a diagnosis The most accurate test is endoscopy (see Tests section, p.68), where a tiny camera on a thin, flexible fiberoptic tube is inserted through the mouth then the esophagus and stomach, examining the tissues on the way. Barium X-ray is sometimes used; in that test, barium is swallowed to coat the lining of the digestive tract and make the esophagus and stomach more visible on the X-ray (see Tests section, p.66). Another test that may be required is a pH probe to measure acid levels in the esophagus.

NORMAL

Gastroesophageal valve
tightly shut, keeping stomach
contents secure

Diaphragm

REFLUX

Gastroesophageal
valve open

Acidic stomach
contents leak back
into esophagus

Gastroesophageal reflux occurs when the acidic stomach contents leak back into the esophagus, causing heartburn symptoms. This happens when the valve at the top of the stomach fails to remain tightly closed.

Strategies for managing GERD There are a number of steps you can take to improve the symptoms of GERD.

Avoiding foods and beverages that can weaken the LES is recommended. These include chocolate, peppermint, fatty foods, coffee, and alcoholic beverages. Foods and beverages that can irritate a damaged esophageal lining (such as citrus fruits and juices, tomato products, and chilli) should also be avoided. Also, because fatty foods delay the stomach's emptying of its contents into the duodenum, intake of these foods should be reduced.

Decreasing the size of portions at mealtime may also help control symptoms. Eating meals at least 2–3 hours before bedtime may lessen reflux by allowing the acid in the stomach to decrease and the stomach to empty partially. In addition, being overweight often worsens symptoms. Many overweight people find relief when they lose weight.

Cigarette smoking weakens the LES. Therefore, stopping smoking is important in reducing GERD symptoms.

A diet high in fiber may ease the symptoms of an ulcer or nonulcer dyspepsia, but you should also cut down on aggravating factors, such as smoking.

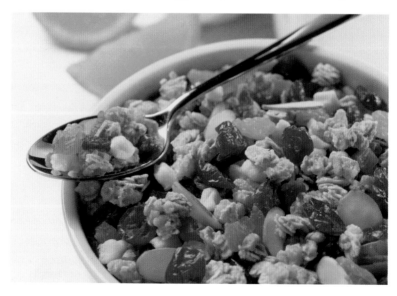

Elevating the head of the bed on 3–6 in (7.5–15 cm) blocks or sleeping on a specially designed wedge reduces heartburn by allowing gravity to minimize reflux of stomach contents into the esophagus.

Antacids may be helpful for occasional or mild heartburn. They neutralize gastric acid and provide quick temporary relief, but long-term use can result in adverse effects. These include diarrhea, altered calcium metabolism (a change in the way the body breaks down and uses calcium) and, rarely, a buildup of magnesium in the body. Too much magnesium can be serious for patients with kidney disease. If antacids are needed for more than 2 weeks, you should consult your doctor.

Your doctor may prescribe acid-blocking drugs. These include cimetidine (Tagamet) and ranitidine (Zantac). The most effective medication currently prescribed is omeprazole (Prilosec). These proton pump inhibitors block acid production and allow the damaged esophageal tissues time to heal. These drugs are usually well tolerated for long-term use. Sometimes drugs that increase gastric emptying are also prescribed.

Although there are no well-researched natural remedies for use in GERD, some herbalists and naturopaths prescribe deglycyrrhizinated licorice (DGL), which has a good track record in helping to heal stomach ulcers, in addition to giving lifestyle and dietary guidance. Chewable lozenges may be the best form to take to relieve GERD.

GERD is common in pregnancy, especially in the third trimester. Chewable papaya tablets may provide relief and are safe for pregnant women.

Surgery may be required if you have a large hiatal hernia. This occurs when the upper stomach pushes through the opening in the diaphragm where the esophagus passes. Mostly these produce no symptoms at all, but if the hernia is sufficiently large it may displace the sphincter and allow acid to reach the esophagus. Surgery may also be used to improve the functioning of the sphincter.

Ulcers and stomach pain

Peptic ulcers are another common cause of indigestion, although less common than gastroesophageal reflux. There are two types of peptic ulcers—gastric ulcers, which occur in the stomach and duodenal ulcers, which develop in the first part of the small intestine. The most common symptom of a peptic ulcer is gnawing pain in the

THE PAIN OF A PEPTIC ULCER:

- can be a dull, gnawing ache or a sharp, stabbing pain.
- can come and go for several days or weeks.
- can occur $1/2$–3 hours after a meal.
- can occur in the middle of the night (when the stomach is empty).
- can be relieved by some foods and beverages (such as milk).

upper abdomen. The pain is caused by stomach acid washing over an open sore. Food may buffer the acid and sometimes eating temporarily relieves the pain. Other signs and symptoms include weight loss, poor appetite, vomiting, bloating, belching, and midback pain. The open sore may lead to internal bleeding and vomiting of blood (which may look like coffee grounds) or very dark, tarry stools that have blood in them.

The stomach wall is protected against the acidic stomach secretions by a thick mucus lining. The duodenum is protected against acid by neutralizing factors as well as by a rapid replacement of the cells that make up the intestinal wall. This ensures that the surface in contact with the acid is always renewed. Normally this will be enough to ensure that an ulcer does not form. However, there are various factors that can weaken these protective mechanisms. It is now well established that the bacterium *Helicobacter pylori* is found in more than 75 percent of patients with gastric ulcers and more than 90 percent of those with duodenal ulcers. Antibiotic treatment is quite successful in these cases. There are, however, other important factors that damage the stomach and duodenal lining. Alcohol and nonsteroidal anti-inflammatory drugs, such as aspirin and ibuprofen, can cause ulcers. Smoking increases the production of stomach acid and delays healing when an ulcer forms.

Nonulcer dyspepsia Ulcers and GERD are not the only important causes of indigestion. Nonulcer dyspepsia is a common diagnosis made only by ruling out other conditions. It is important to be sure that there is not an ulcer, because the complications from ulcers can be serious, such as intractable pain, hemorrhage, perforation, or obstruction. If tests fail to reveal an ulcer or GERD, you may be evaluated for gallstones, liver or pancreatic disease, or irritable bowel syndrome— all of which can produce symptoms of indigestion.

Hypochlorhydria Sometimes dyspepsia occurs when stomach acid levels are low. Although these levels tend to decrease with age, there are differences of opinion as to how prevalent hypochloridia is; some studies have shown that nearly half of those over age 60 have low levels of stomach acidity. There are various diseases associated with low gastric acidity, the most well-known being pernicious anemia. Low acid output predisposes the stomach to *H. pylori* colonization, so paradoxically in some cases ulcers are precipitated by low rather than high acid levels. Common signs and symptoms include belching, a burning sensation immediately after meals, a feeling that the food just sits in the stomach without digesting, and the inability to eat more than small amounts at a time. Low levels of hydrochloric acid can lead to bacteria and parasites passing through the stomach into the intestines and causing infection. Proteins that are insufficiently broken down by stomach acid can lead to allergies if they pass through the intestinal wall. The definitive test is a gastric capsule analysis, in which a capsule that transmits radio signals is swallowed and measures the acid levels. The procedure for this test is described in the Tests section (p.69). If the symptoms strongly suggest hypochlorhydria, betaine hydrochloride supplements may be taken with caution (see p.43).

Nonulcer dyspepsia may be distressing but is never a serious medical condition; however, before embarking on self-treatment you should always have appropriate medical diagnosis if your symptoms are severe or persistent.

Establishing a diagnosis In an endoscopy, a thin flexible tube with a tiny camera on the end is inserted in the patient's mouth and swallowed down the throat, in order to examine the esophagus, stomach, and duodenum. The camera takes pictures, and small tissue samples can be taken to view under a microscope.

H. pylori may be tested for in several ways, including blood, saliva, breath, biopsy samples, and endoscopy. Each test has its specific uses.

Therapeutics First try and identify and eliminate or cut down on the factors that are known to contribute toward ulcers and nonulcer dyspepsia. First among these is alcohol and anti-inflammatory drugs. You should stop taking these if you have an ulcer. If that is not possible, then taking them with food may lessen their irritant effect. Smoking increases stomach acid production and delays healing, so eliminating or cutting down will help. A fiber-rich diet is both protective and may be used therapeutically.

The significance of stress in peptic ulcers is controversial. Although animal and human studies demonstrate that extreme stress leads to ulcers, comparable studies have not convincingly demonstrated that peptic ulcer patients suffer any more stress than those who do not suffer from ulcers. The crucial factor is likely to be how individuals respond to stress.

Mainstream medicine A combination of antibiotics to kill *H. pylori* and acid-suppressing medication or proton pump inhibitors is the mainstay of the medical approach—and has proved effective in eliminating *H. pylori* and allowing ulcers to heal. For nonulcer dyspepsia, acid-suppressing medications and antibiotics are usually ineffective. If adjusting diet and lifestyle does not bring sufficient relief, your doctor may prescribe such drugs as domperidone or metoclopramide to alter the way the stomach empties itself.

Complementary and alternative therapeutics
■ Deglycrrhizinated Licorice (DGL) DGL is an excellent antiulcer preparation from which the glycyrrhetinic acid is removed. This avoids the potential adverse effects of fluid retention and raised blood pressure, which can come from long-term use of crude licorice preparations. DGL is free from adverse effects, but its safety has not

been evaluated during pregnancy. Chewable tablets are the most effective for peptic ulcers, because DGL needs to mix with saliva. The standard dose is two to four 400-mg chewable tablets between meals or 20 minutes before meals.

■ **Cabbage juice** has a reputation for helping to heal ulcers. See Juicing (p.104) in Options for Health: Simple Remedies.

■ **Bismuth Chelate** (tripotassium dicitratobismuthate) (120 mg four times a day for 8 weeks) may be helpful in eradicating *H. pylori* and reducing the recurrence of peptic ulcer disease. Combining it with barberry (*Berberis vulgaris*), goldenseal (*Hydrastis canadensis*), or Oregon grape (*Berberis aquifolium*) may strengthen its antimicrobial effects. Take it alone or in a combination tincture. The dose is 2 ml three times a day. Taking bismuth preparations may temporarily darken the tongue and feces.

■ **Hypochlorhydria (insufficient stomach acid)** The protocol for supplementing with hydrochloric acid (HC1) is as follows: Start by taking one tablet containing 600 mg of HC1 with a large meal. If this does not aggravate the symptoms, increase the dosage at each meal to a maximum of seven tablets until you feel a warmth in your stomach. This indicates you have taken more HC1 than needed for that meal. Reduce the dosage by one tablet at your next meal. When you establish the largest dose you can take at one meal without the feeling of warmth, maintain the dose for all meals of a similar size. You should take less for smaller meals. The tablets are best taken spread throughout the meal. As your stomach regains the ability to produce sufficient HC1, you will notice the warm feeling, and you should reduce the dosage accordingly. This is not a generally accepted conventional medical treatment, but many naturopaths and some nutritionally oriented doctors find the protocol useful for nonulcer dyspepsia.

Food allergies may be implicated, and an elimination diet may be helpful for recurrent problems (see allergy and immunity on p.69 of Tests).

Parasites and other infections

Many people associate parasitic infections with travel to foreign countries, but there are numerous sources of infectious food and drinks close to home, in spite of modern sanitation and water treatment. In addition to home-grown microorganisms, increased overseas travel and food importation has brought more people into

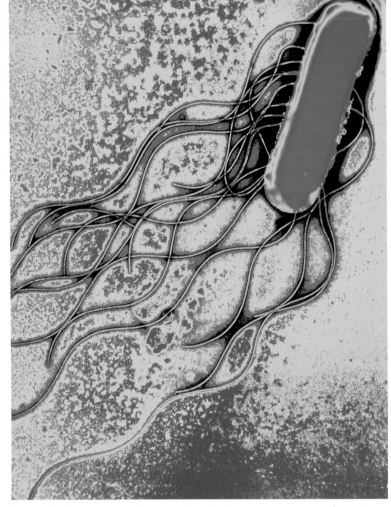

Salmonella is a genus of microorganism that is a common cause of parasitic infection or food poisoning. Usually the symptoms of stomach upset will pass within a couple of days. If not, consult your doctor without delay.

contact with exotic microorganisms. The illnesses resulting from infection range from simple stomach upsets to more serious signs and symptoms, including diarrhea, fever, vomiting, abdominal cramps, and dehydration. Sometimes, in susceptible individuals, chronic infection can trigger arthritis, inflammatory bowel disease, and autoimmune disorders, in which the immune system attacks the body's own cells. General signs and symptoms (such as weight loss, fatigue, muscular and joint pain, and allergies) may also be the result of chronic intestinal infections.

Although sound food and personal hygiene are important in preventing the spread of infectious microorganisms, it is extremely difficult to avoid contact with these potential pathogens. There are many sources of infection, such as food, water, personal contact, and pets.

The list of possible infectious organisms is extensive and includes bacteria, protozoa, amoebae, and worms of various kinds (roundworm, pinworm, hookworm). Among the most common pathogens are *Escherichia coli*, *Salmonella* sp., *Entamoeba histolytica*, *Helicobacter pylori* (see Ulcers and stomach pain on p.39), *Blastocystis hominis*, *Giardia lamblia*, and *Cryptosporidium* sp.

Diagnosis Accurate diagnosis of parasitic infections can be extremely difficult. Stool samples are taken at 2- or 4-day intervals. Repeated testing may be required to establish a diagnosis, because the organisms may not be detectable in every stool sample. Finding the organism causing dysentery may be difficult, because organisms such as *Giardia* adhere tightly to the small intestine wall and may not be detected unless the stool sample is from a bout of diarrhea or use of a purgative when material from the small intestine will be found in the feces.

Treatment Bacterial infection with salmonella or *E. coli* in an otherwise healthy adult will usually pass after a couple of days of digestive upset. In those who are very young or old and in those with an impaired immune system, these infections are more serious and require careful supervision. Some microorganisms (such as *Listeria monocytogenes* and *Clostridium botulinum*) cause far more serious illness than vomiting or diarrhea. Although uncommon, they can cause spontaneous abortion or death. Infection in these cases is a medical emergency.

Infections with amoebae, worms, or giardia will require specific antibiotics. It is important that these infections are treated vigorously and that the course of antibiotics is completed, because partially treated infections may mean that antibiotic-resistant strains develop and the infection becomes more deep-seated.

Herbs that can help Herbs containing berberine, such as goldenseal (hydrastis canadensis) have been shown to be effective in research studies in eliminating a wide range of infectious organisms in the gastrointestinal tract and may be a good adjunct to antibiotic treatment. It makes good sense to use supplements containing the beneficial bacteria that normally inhabit the gut, such as *Lactobacillus acidophilus*, and bifidobacteria. The amino acid L-glutamine can help heal an irritated gut lining resulting from infection.

Dysbiosis

The healthy gut is host to a wide variety of bacteria. Many hundreds have been identified as transient visitors, but only a handful are found in large quantities. They all form part of a complex microecology through which the body maintains balance. The friendly bacteria assist in digestion, produce essential vitamins, and detoxify undigested products in the diet. There are also unwelcome visitors, which, if they gain a foothold, may produce, for example, gastroenteritis, vitamin deficiencies, and toxins. Dysbiosis is a condition in which the microbiological balance is upset and functioning ineffectively. This condition can lead to disease, rather than being a specific disease itself, and is generally not a term that conventional practitioners use.

Although several factors can disturb the microecology of the bowel, the most important is the use of antibiotics. As well as eliminating bacterial infections, antibiotics also have a dramatic effect on beneficial bacteria. This is especially true of two of the most important friendly bacteria, *Lactobacillus acidophilus* and bifidobacteria, which are particularly sensitive to a wide range of antibiotics. A healthy gut can usually recover after a single course of antibiotics, but repeated courses make it difficult to restore the normal balance. The reduction in the beneficial flora makes the gut prone to opportunistic pathogens and overgrowth by antibiotic-resistant flora, such as *E. coli* and *Candida albicans*, both of which are normally held in check by lactobacilli and bifidobacteria. Fiber is a major source of nutrition for the friendly flora. A low-fiber diet is insufficient to support the optimal balance of flora. Corticosteroids, nonsteroidal anti-inflammatory drugs (NSAIDs), and stress have also been implicated in disturbing gut function and promoting dysbiosis.

The symptoms of dysbiosis Bloating, constipation, diarrhea, fatigue, and flatulence are common signs and symptoms of dysbiosis. Some people have increased sensitivity to foods and the environment, with additional symptoms of skin problems and some forms of arthritis. This type of dysbiosis is often associated with leaky gut and food allergy.

Diagnosis The diagnosis of dysbiosis is mainly made by nutritionally oriented doctors or naturopaths. Many conventionally trained doctors are unfamiliar with the condition, however, research is growing to support the diagnosis. The symptoms and medical history are suggestive, and a comprehensive digestive stool analysis (see Tests, p.65) is used to establish whether the intestinal flora is adequately balanced. Again, this test is not widely used by conventional practitioners.

Treatment A diet based on plant fiber provides the substrate on which beneficial flora thrive. Oat fiber, soy, banana, and onions are rich in fructooligosaccharides, providing food for the beneficial bacteria.

Supplementation with *Lactobacillus acidophilus* and bifidobacteria helps recolonize the gut and should always be used after a course of antibiotics. It is important to take a sufficient amount of a high-quality supplement to be effective. Doses containing at least one billion viable organisms are recommended. The organisms are easily destroyed by variations in temperature and, depending on the method used for drying and encapsulation, may require refrigeration. Choose a reputable brand, and follow the directions for storage and use.

CONDITIONS ASSOCIATED WITH LEAKY GUT

- Autoimmune conditions: ankylosing spondylitis, rheumatoid arthritis, psoriatic arthritis
- Gastrointestinal conditions: gastroenteritis, ulcerative colitis, pancreatitis
- Skin conditions: eczema, urticaria, psoriasis
- Some cases of asthma, food and environmental allergies, chronic fatigue syndrome

Leaky gut syndrome

Leaky gut syndrome is a term used by nutritionally oriented doctors and naturopaths to describe a state of increased intestinal permeability. Doctors of conventional medicine are probably unfamiliar with the syndrome. Leaky gut is a process that can lead to disease rather than being a specific disease itself. The gut has to balance two opposing functions. First, it balances the absorption of nutrients, and second, it acts as a barrier to microbes and large undigested food particles by preventing their entry into the bloodstream. The tight junctions that exist between the lining cells of the intestines limits the passage of molecules. When larger molecules pass through the gut wall, an immune response may be triggered and inflammation may result as white cells engulf the foreign substances. The inflammation that the immune response causes also increases the permeability of the gut wall, thus perpetuating this vicious circle. Disruption of these tight junctions occurs for various reasons, including inflammation, damage to the gut by NSAIDs, gastrointestinal infections, and dysbiosis. Such distruption is also a result of bowel diseases such as celiac disease and Crohn's disease.

The number of conditions associated with increased intestinal permeability grows as more is understood about the relationship between the digestive system and immunity, but it is not always clear whether these are causes or effects.

Increased absorption of foreign substances increases the demand on the liver. The liver is the great detoxifier of the body. All substances absorbed across the intestinal barrier pass through the liver before entering the general circulation. The liver has a remarkable reserve capacity, but eventually this capacity may be exceeded and toxic substances pass into the general circulation and create problems throughout the body. As time goes on, those with leaky gut tend to become more sensitive to food and environmental substances.

Diagnosis The significance of leaky gut syndrome has not been widely recognized in conventional medicine, although research underpinning the link between leaky gut and a range of health problems is increasing. A simple intestinal absorption test can help establish whether there is increased intestinal permeability. A large molecule sugar mixture is administered and the degree of absorption is measured from the urine after 6 hours. This test is performed by laboratories specializing in nutritional medicine and may not be widely available. A comprehensive digestive stool analysis (CDSA) and parasitology tests may be helpful in establishing the cause of the leaky gut.

Managing leaky gut The key is removal of factors known to cause the condition. Substances that irritate or inflame the gut wall (such as NSAIDs and alcohol) should be avoided. If dysbiosis is present, that must be addressed. Supplements such as the amino acid L-glutamine can help the gut lining to repair.

Refer to dysbiosis on p.46, and parasites and other infections on p.43. Also see intestinal permeability (p.66), and CDSA (p.65) in Tests.

Food allergies and intolerance

The relationship between certain foods and digestive problems is well recognized, but not all adverse reactions are classed as food allergies. In some individuals, foods containing histamine (fish) or tyramine (some cheeses or red wines) can have a drug-like (pharmacological) action and trigger an inflammatory response. This can lead to allergy-like signs and symptoms, such as skin rashes, migraines, and gut problems.

Some people cannot tolerate gluten in wheat and other grains and are afflicted with a malabsorption problem called celiac disease (see p.55). A common cause of intolerance to dairy food is a deficiency of lactase, which is the enzyme necessary to digest the sugar found in milk. These reactions have been described as intolerances or sensitivities. Within medicine the term *allergy* is reserved for those reactions to food or environment that trigger an immunological response.

Food and the immune system Food presents an enormous challenge to the immune system, and the gut is the largest organ of immunity in the body. Every day you take into your body various foreign substances, known as antigens, that the digestive system has broken down for absorption. With normal health, only a small amount of foreign substances pass through the gut wall, and these antigens are dealt with by the immune cells located along the intestinal tract. If the gut wall becomes more permeable to foreign proteins, the body will mount a more general immune response.

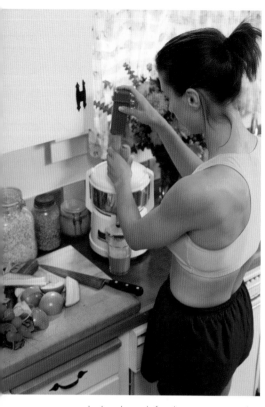

If you can maintain the motivation to see it through, an oral food challenge, or elimination diet, may be the best way to discover if you have a food allergy.

The classic type I allergic response is where an immediate hypersensitivity is demonstrated. This reaction is responsible for the typical symptoms of hay fever, hives, and asthma. The immune system produces antibodies to the foreign particle, or antigen, which then bind with it and triggers swelling and inflammation. The antibodies responsible for these immediate reactions are known as IgE (Ig means immunoglobulin and E describes the class). The body's response is strong and clear-cut, and symptoms can occur within seconds to minutes after exposure, whether through food, contact, or airborne particles. There is an inherited tendency for these kind of allergic responses, although the reaction to specific foods is not inherited. Type I allergic reactions account for only a small percentage of adverse reactions to food. When extreme, the reactions are serious and even life-threatening. The allergic reaction can lead to swelling of the throat or bronchospasm, which blocks the airways. People with this condition need to carry adrenaline with them in case of emergency.

In type II reactions, another class of antibodies (known as IgG) latch onto the foreign particles (antigens) that pass through the gut wall. The immune system then breaks down these foreign particles for removal. If the exposure is not excessive and the immune system is healthy, this process does not provoke symptoms. High levels of the foreign substances passing through the gut wall or an overreaction by the immune system may lead to allergic symptoms.

A type III reaction is where the foreign particles and immune cells that have attached to them are not cleared from the body. These immune complexes are then deposited in various tissues of the body, such as the joints or blood vessels, where they damage the tissues and may lead to symptoms such as arthritis.

Because the response of IgG antibodies is delayed, it may be difficult to establish whether a specific food is responsible for the allergy. The symptoms may not become apparent until some hours or even a day or two after ingestion. The symptoms range from mild to severe.

The symptoms of food intolerance Adverse reactions to food may be far-reaching and may manifest throughout the body systems, affecting immunity (chronic infections), the musculoskeletal system (joint pain, arthritis), the skin (acne, eczema), the respiratory system (asthma, chronic infections), and neurological system (anxiety, depression). The specific digestive problems associated with food intolerance include chronic diarrhea, constipation, malabsorption, and irritable bowel syndrome. Inflammatory bowel diseases, such as Crohn's disease, and ulcerative colitis may also be aggravated by food allergy.

Diagnosing food allergy There is a lack of universally accepted diagnostic criteria for food intolerance. If you suspect a food allergy, the definitive test is the oral food challenge. Reliable laboratory tests are available for type I IgE reactions, although these account for only a small number of adverse reactions to foods. IgG testing is available, but the correlation between raised IgG levels to a specific food and clinical symptoms has not been firmly established. Some practitioners use IgG testing as a guide, but neither IgG nor IgE picks up nonimmunological responses, such as the druglike actions described at the beginning of the chapter. The oral food challenge is the most reliable method for detecting adverse reactions to foods.

Oral food challenge Food challenge is where all suspect food is avoided for a period of time and then reintroduced to see if symptoms are triggered. Although the oral food challenge has the advantage of being without financial cost, the challenge requires a high level of motivation to maintain the adjustments in diet. In practice, all suspect foods are avoided for at least a week. The elimination diet consists of food items least likely to trigger an allergic response, such as rice, bananas, and vegetables such as broccoli and cauliflower. Lamb and pear are known to be well tolerated. If the offending food has been avoided, then the symptoms should begin to clear over a week. One of the foods is then reintroduced each day, and a careful record is made of any returning symptoms. It is not unusual for a hightened sensitivity to occur while on this elimination diet, and the reaction to offending foods may be quite dramatic. When done methodically, this diet is the most reliable method for determining food intolerances and allergies. If no reaction can be detected, this establishes that foods eaten during the elimination phase were not the offending items. If necessary, you should repeat the procedure; however, you should only undertake an elimination diet under medical supervision.

See allergy and immunity in Tests (p.69), and also refer to the dietary advice on pp.76–91) of Lifestyle Changes in Options for Health.

Irritable bowel syndrome

Irritable bowel syndrome (IBS) is a common disorder of the intestines in which bowel habit is altered (diarrhea or constipation), with or without pain. It is typically accompanied by discomfort, gassiness, and bloating and less frequently by the passage of mucus in stools. It has in the past been known by various names, such as spastic colon, mucous colitis, and spastic colitis. The term *syndrome* refers to the fact that no identifiable disease process in the gut can be identified. What is found is a change in the way the gut functions. There is no permanent damage to the intestines, nor is there any resulting bleeding or serious diseases, such as cancer. However, although there may be no detectable disease in the tissues, the condition may be far from trivial for those afflicted. For some sufferers, the condition causes great distress on their social and work lives. This is due mainly to having to respond to the compelling urge for a bowel movement, thereby limiting travel, even over short distances.

What causes IBS The condition affects at least 10 percent of the population, although for many people the condition is mild, so they do not seek medical treatment but manage as best they can with self-help. Women are affected more than men, and the incidence declines with age. There seems to be a relationship with food allergies and stress is a major factor in IBS. Gastrointestinal infection may precipitate IBS.

A key factor in IBS is that the colon is hypersensitive to stimulation. A low level of stimulation affects the gut motility (peristaltic contractions), leading to the characteristic symptoms of IBS—changes in bowel movements, bloating and pain, or discomfort. For someone with IBS, ordinary events (such as eating) and distention from gas or stool in the colon can cause the colon to overreact. Certain medicines and foods may trigger spasms in some people as can anxiety and stress. Sometimes the spasm delays the passage of stool, leading to constipation. Chocolate, dairy products, or large amounts of alcohol are common offenders. Caffeine causes loose stools in many people, but it is more likely to affect those with IBS. Researchers also have found that women with IBS may have more symptoms during their menstrual periods, suggesting that reproductive hormones may exacerbate IBS symptoms.

The potential for abnormal function of the colon is always present in people with IBS, but a trigger also must be present to cause symptoms. The most likely culprits are diet, a disordered gut ecology (dysbiosis), and emotional stress.

Diagnosis Diagnosis depends on a complete medical history, careful description of the symptoms, and a physical examination to rule out other conditions. Although there are no specific tests for IBS, blood, stool, urine, and endoscopy tests are sometimes required to rule out other diseases. The comprehensive digestive stool analysis may be helpful in diagnosing dysbiosis.

Managing IBS For many people, eating a proper diet and managing stress effectively lessens IBS symptoms. Before changing your diet, it is a good idea to keep a journal noting which foods seem to cause distress. Discuss your findings with your health care provider. A nutritionist, naturopath, or nutritionally oriented doctor will help you make changes in your diet and arrange tests if food allergy is suspected.

Fiber: A double-edged sword Fiber may be both a cause and cure of symptoms. High-fiber diets keep the colon slightly distended, which may help to prevent spasms from developing. By softening and speeding the passage of stool, high-fiber diets reduce constipation, but for some people, the fiber in wheat also leads to an increase of diarrhea, gas, and pain. The insoluble wheat fiber ferments in the colon, and the gases given off create colon distention. Wheat bran is a common source of insoluble fiber, but wheat is also a common allergen. All plant food contains fiber—not just whole grains and bran. The fiber in fruit, vegetables, pulses, and oats is water soluble and produces a softer stool that is easier to pass and gentler on the colon. Because increasing fiber in the diet can cause gas and bloating, make the changes gradually over a few weeks, until the body is accustomed to the new diet.

Large meals can cause cramping and diarrhea in people with IBS. Symptoms may be eased if you eat smaller meals more often or just eat smaller portions. However, if constipation is the main problem, medium to large meals are more effective at stimulating the peristaltic movement of the bowel. The bowel is a creature of habit and eating regular meals helps to establish a regular pattern of bowel movement. Some people are helped by avoiding fatty foods, beans and other gas-

A high-fiber diet can exacerbate or alleviate the symptoms of IBS.

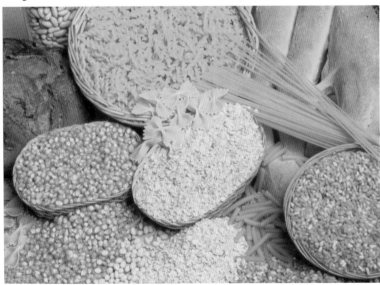

producing foods, and alcohol and caffeine, which can irritate the intestines. Drink plenty of fluids to prevent constipation—water is best. Alcohol and beverages that contain caffeine have a diuretic effect, so the fluid is passed out through the urine rather than being reabsorbed into the stool. Carbonated drinks should be avoided because these create extra gas and bloating in the digestive system. Some people cannot tolerate the milk sugar lactose and should avoid or strictly limit dairy products. The undigested lactose passes into the colon where bacteria use it as a source of food, and in doing so produce a large amount of uncomfortable gas.

For further information, see the dietary advice on pp.76–85 of Lifestyle Changes in Options for Health.

Stress Many people with IBS recognize that stress makes their symptoms worse: When the symptoms increase stress levels, there is a corresponding worsening of the symptoms. An important step in controlling IBS is learning how to effectively deal with stress. Learning a relaxation exercise can be useful, and there are many from which to choose. The section on managing stress describes some of these. There is good evidence that hypnosis can be helpful in controlling the symptoms of IBS. Exercise is an important part of a stress management strategy, and it helps regulate the peristaltic wave through the gut.

See relaxing and managing stress on p.92, and exercise on p.98, of Lifestyle Changes in Options for Health.

Medication A water-soluble fiber supplement can be taken in the form of oat bran, psyllium seed husks, or flaxseed. Artichoke extract is very helpful in relieving bloating, loss of appetite, nausea, and the abdominal pain associated with IBS. Peppermint oil capsules have a relaxant effect on the intestinal muscles and are quite effective in reducing the symptoms of IBS; however, the capsules should be enteric-coated, to prevent the oil from being released in the stomach where it can cause heartburn.

Celiac disease

People with celiac disease have an immunological reaction to gluten. It damages the tiny projections in the small intestine called villi and interferes with their ability to absorb certain nutrients. The disease affects children and adults. At least 1 in 1,000 people—and in some populations as many as 1 in 200 people—have the disease. The effects in children are diarrhea, growth failure, and failure to thrive. Symptoms may also be detected in adults, but because the symptoms can be vague, they are usually attributed to other conditions, such as IBS. Signs and symptoms can include bloating, diarrhea, abdominal pain, skin rash, anemia, and osteoporosis. Celiac disease may cause such nonspecific signs and symptoms for several years before being correctly diagnosed and treated. The first step in diagnosis is to check the blood for antibodies to gluten. These are called antigliadin antibodies. If test results are positive and the symptoms suggest celiac disease, a small tissue sample (biopsy) may be taken with an endoscope to confirm the diagnosis.

People with celiac disease must avoid foods containing gluten, which is a protein in wheat, rye, barley, and possibly oats, regardless of whether they have symptoms. In these people, gluten destroys part of the lining of the small intestine, which interferes with the absorption of nutrients. The damage can occur from even a small amount of gluten, and not everyone has symptoms of damage.

Inflammatory bowel disease

Under the general heading of inflammatory bowel disease (IBD) are two main conditions, Crohn's disease and ulcerative colitis. IBD involves inflammation of the digestive tract anywhere from the mouth to the rectum. The causes are not clearly understood, but there is evidence of a range of influences, from genetic to dietary. IBD may cause diffuse symptoms, and diagnosis may be difficult to establish. People with IBD are at somewhat greater risk for cancer.

Crohn's disease is characterized by inflammatory changes in the colon, small intestine, or any other part of the digestive tract. The person with Crohn's has bouts of diarrhea and low-grade fever. Pain and tenderness in the right lower abdomen is likely to be present, and the person may also experience constipation. Over time, the person may lose weight due to reduced appetite and poor absorption of nutrients. Diagnosis is confirmed by colonoscopy and biopsy.

Ulcerative colitis is more common, and the inflammation is mostly confined to the lining of the colon. Common signs and symptoms are bloody diarrhea with cramps and abdominal tenderness, but there may also be constipation. Weight loss is less common than in Crohn's disease, and diagnosis is confirmed by colonoscopy and biopsy.

Both Crohn's disease and ulcerative colitis share many common features and will be discussed together as variants of IBD. There is a genetic predisposition to IBD, and some close relatives are likely to suffer from it. People of European descent have a higher incidence of IBD, and Irish and Jewish populations are at much greater risk. The onset may be at any age, but it is most common between ages 15 and 35.

The suggested causes include infection by viruses and autoimmune reactions. There is some evidence to show that diet may be an important influence, not only in the onset of the disease but also in its ongoing management. Foods like wheat and dairy can be triggers, so removing allergens from the diet may modify the course of IBD. (See food allergies and intolerance on p.49.) Changes in intestinal permeability have been shown to precede flare-ups of IBD. Increased permeability of the gut allows allergens to enter the body, and this permeability is increased through the use of anti-inflammatory drugs and infection by parasites.

Some naturopaths and nutritionally oriented doctors recommend avoiding foods that can cause inflammation, such as red meat and dairy, and increasing consumption of cold-water fish such as salmon, mackerel, and herring, which are rich in omega-3 fatty acids, to help modulate the inflammatory response. Obtaining all your nutrients is important, so you should take a good multivitamin and mineral supplement. Deficiencies are known to occur in IBD, and a sufficient intake of zinc, vitamin B_{12}, and folic acid is particularly important.

The mainstream approach to treatment is based on medication, and in extremely severe cases surgery may be required. Medications include anti-inflammatory drugs and corticosteroids to reduce inflammation and suppress the immune system. Many of these medications have adverse effects, including increasing the permeability of the gut wall to allergens, but the severity of the condition may require their use.

Naturopathy (see p.130), herbal medicine (see p.126), and homeopathy (see p.128) have a place in the treatment of bowel diseases, even if only in a supportive capacity, and they may sometimes improve the symptoms significantly.

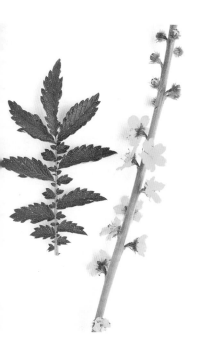

Preparations using common agrimony can increase bile production and treat jaundice, other liver diseases, and skin complaints.

Diverticular disease

Diverticula are small pouches that form in the digestive tract and most commonly affect the lower bowel. They do not normally cause symptoms, and most people only discover they have the condition following examination for other problems, such as screening for bowel cancer. The presence of diverticula is known as diverticulosis. Any inflammation that develops within the pouches is called diverticulitis. The inflammation causes pain (most commonly in the left lower abdomen), changes in bowel habit, fever and nausea. The condition is usually serious and should be evaluated by a health care professional.

The main cause of diverticular disease is a low-fiber diet. The condition is virtually unknown in populations that do not eat refined flour and grains. Insufficient fiber leads to small hard stools, which are difficult to pass. Aging thickens the bowel wall, making the passage of stool through the bowel more difficult. Straining to pass these stools puts pressure on the weakest points in the muscle of the intestinal wall. This results in ballooning of the weakened areas and causes the pouches that lead to diverticulitis.

If no symptoms are apparent, self-care should be based on increasing the fiber content of the diet and avoiding constipation. You should consume 25–30 grams of fiber as part of your daily diet. The fiber from fruit, vegetables, legumes, and oats is soluble and absorbs up to fifteen times its weight in water, which softens the stool. Insoluble fiber from wheat, rice, and corn adds bulk and encourages the passage of the stool. If you find it difficult to achieve a sufficient fiber intake, consider using a supplement such as psyllium husks or cracked linseed (flaxseed). Simply remember to increase your fluid intake when you increase your fiber intake, otherwise the fiber can have a constipating effect.

Refer to the text on diarrhea and constipation on pp.30–33 of Signs and Symptoms, and the dietary advice on pp.76–91 of Lifestyle Changes in Options for Health.

Gallbladder and liver disease

Gallstones and cholecystitis The liver and gallbladder contribute to digestion in several important ways. There are many tasks that the liver performs, including filtering and processing chemicals in food, storing nutrients, and breaking down old blood cells. The liver produces bile as a waste product of chemical processes in the liver, but bile also assists in the digestion of fats by breaking the fat globules down to a manageable size for the fat digestive enzymes. Bile also helps eliminate wastes from the blood and promotes the incorporation of water into the stool. Without enough bile, the stool can become hard and difficult to pass.

While the liver goes on secreting bile into the duodenum, the gallbladder stores and concentrates bile for use when fats are eaten. If bile becomes too concentrated for use, stonelike formations occur within the gallbladder. These consist of varying proportions of cholesterol, pigment, and calcium. Gallstones are common and in most people do not cause symptoms. If they become lodged within the bile duct, the flow of bile into the duodenum is blocked and the gallbladder may become inflamed. The main symptoms are attacks of upper abdominal pain. The pain may be displaced into the back, chest, or right shoulder blade, or it may be very severe and accompanied by nausea and vomiting. Attacks may be triggered by eating fatty foods, but if the blockage is only partial and there is little inflammation, bloating and a dull ache after meals may be the only symptoms.

A diet high in fats and sugar combined with a sedentary lifestyle increases the risk of gallstones. Although they are more common in women who are fair skinned and who have had children, and who tend to carry excess weight, rapid weight loss diets also increase the risk of stone formation by altering bile chemistry.

Diagnosis is by ultrasound or scan, and if gallstones are found but you have never had symptoms, the best advice is to gradually achieve your optimum weight by reducing your intake of fats and sugars, increasing your intake of fiber, and exercising regularly. Food allergens may irritate the gallbladder. If the gallstones are predominantly made up of cholesterol, prescription medications can help to dissolve them, although they recur in about one in four persons. There are several complementary treatments that may offer a long-term strategy for reducing and preventing gallstones. Enteric-coated peppermint oil capsules can help dissolve some gallstones. Herbs such as milk thistle (*Silybum marianum*) and dandelion root (*Taraxicum officinalis*) stimulate bile production and solubility. A nutrient such as lecithin emulsifies cholesterol and facilitates its secretion.

Hepatitis The most common liver disease is hepatitis (inflammation of the liver). This may be induced by alcohol or drugs and can also be the result of viral infections. The symptoms may point to a digestive disorder with loss of appetite, nausea, fatigue, unexplained weight loss, and yellowing of the skin (jaundice).

The infection may be transmitted via contaminated food or water in hepatitis A, which is the least serious form of hepatitis and mostly resolves with treatment. More serious are hepatitis B, which is transmitted by blood, semen, and saliva, and hepatitis C by blood or blood products. Types D and E are other variants. If the inflammation of the liver becomes chronic (lasts longer than 6 months), scar tissue may form (cirrhosis), leading in some cases to liver failure. There is also a greater risk of liver cancer. The danger with chronic viral hepatitis is that people may have the disease for years without knowing and pass it on to others.

Urine and blood tests are used to diagnose hepatitis. There are no specific medical treatments, but corticosteroids are used to suppress the inflammation and interferon to inhibit the virus from replicating.

Maintaining a healthy lifestyle and avoiding alcohol and drugs assists recovery. Herbs such as milk thistle (*Silybum marianum*) protects the liver and prevents necrotic changes. The antioxidant nutrient alpha-lipoic acid helps prevent cell damage to the liver and assists in its detoxifying functions. Hepatitis is a serious medical condition, and you should seek the advice of your health care provider before taking any herbs or medications to treat its symptoms.

Refer to the dietary advice (What to Eat through to What to Avoid) on pp. 76–91 of Lifestyle Changes in Options for Health.

Cancers of the digestive system

The first thing that must be said is that cancer is not a common cause of

RISK FACTORS FOR COLORECTAL CANCER

The following factors increase the risk of colorectal cancer.

- Heredity: Your risk is increased if other members of your family have colorectal cancer.
- Polyps: Nearly all colorectal cancers start with polyps
- Age: 90 percent of colorectal cancer is in people over age 50.
- Smoking: Smokers have a higher colorectal cancer rate.
- Inflammatory bowel disease: Both ulcerative colitis and Crohn's disease can increase the risk of colorectal cancer.
- Diet: A diet that is high in saturated fat (particularly from red meat such as beef, pork, and lamb) and low in fruit and vegetables is a predisposing factor.
- Exercise: People who are inactive have a somewhat increased risk.

gastrointestinal problems. It is, however, a very serious one, so it is important to recognize its symptoms so they can be dealt with at the earliest possible stage. Signs and symptoms such as bleeding, difficulty swallowing, unexplained weight loss, and a change in bowel habits can be warning signs and should be checked out by a doctor. If cancers are detected and treated early enough, the prognosis is good. The difficulty is that the symptoms are often so vague that the disease is not diagnosed until it reaches an advanced stage.

Cancer is a growth of abnormal cells. As they grow, they form into small tumors that can exert direct pressure on nerves and blood vessels, or interfere with the function of the vital organs—for example, by obstructing the intestines. The growth of some cancers is very slow and can take years for them to become life-threatening, whereas others can grow very rapidly. The cause of cancer seems to be a complex mix of factors, such as lifestyle, environment, and heredity. It is thought that some people have a genetic predisposition toward cancer-producing cells. These genes are activated by an outside agent, possibly an infection, or contact with carcinogens in tobacco or other pollutants in food, the air, or water. Cancers are named according to the type of tissue in which they occur. Carcinomas begin in the tissues of organs, the most common of which are gastrointestinal. Lymphomas develop in the immune system, particularly in the lymph nodes, and sarcomas start in the connective tissue such as muscle or bone.

Colorectal cancer Cancers may occur throughout the digestive tract, but the most common site is the colon and rectum. Colorectal cancer begins with changes in the intestinal lining and the development of polyps. Although not all polyps become cancerous, nearly all colon cancers start as polyps. Screening can help detect colorectal cancer in its early stages. The risk of having colorectal polyps increases with age and as many as four out of ten people over age 60 have polyps. The screening is done with a procedure called a colonoscopy, during which the polyps can be removed. Regular screening should start at age 50 and be repeated every 5 years for high-risk patients. It may be started earlier and repeated more often if you have an increased risk of colorectal cancer. Because the disease may produce no symptoms until it is quite advanced, regular screening can be a lifesaver.

The survival rate for colorectal cancer is very good if diagnosed and treated early. More than 90 percent of people who have their colorectal cancer treated at an early stage exceed the 5-year survival rate.

Other cancers of the digestive tract Cancer can develop anywhere along the espohagus. The cause is not well understood but your risk is increased if you are a smoker, drink alcohol excessively, or suffer from GERD (see p.36). Diets low in fruit and vegetables also increase the risk. The early warnings are:

- difficulty swallowing
- blood in vomit or stool.

The incidence of stomach cancer has decreased over the last 100 years in the US and UK but is still common in Japan. It is believed that this is due to changes in preservation methods of foods. Formerly, salting and smoking food was common, and this process leads to the formation of carcinogens. Infection with *Helicobacter pylori*, which is the bacteria associated with peptic ulcers, also increases the risk of stomach cancer.

Cancer of the liver, gallbladder, bile duct, and pancreas are not common but signs and symptoms such as abdominal pain, yellowing of the skin and eyes (jaundice), abdominal swelling, and weight loss should not be ignored. If you have any of these signs and symptoms, see your doctor immediately.

Unexplained weight loss can be a warning sign of cancer of the esophagus.

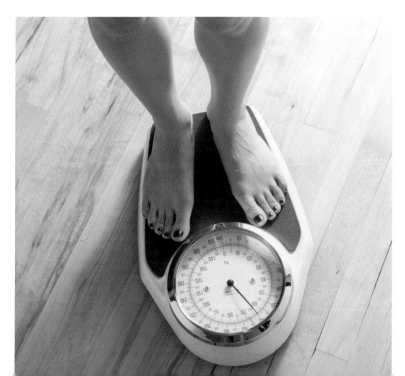

tests for the
digestive
system

There are times, however, when further tests are required to clarify whether symptoms such as abdominal pain are due to irritable bowel syndrome (IBS) or something more sinister such as IBD or cancer. The choice of tests is determined by the severity, persistence, or unusual nature of the symptoms as well as the availability of the test.

Blood

Blood tests provide a great deal of information about how the body is functioning and are generally used because they are relatively simple to perform. A small amount of blood is drawn, either in your health care provider's office or in a specialist's laboratory. If a person has gastrointestinal bleeding and has become anemic, this will show on the complete blood count. An increase in the white blood cell count can indicate the body's immune response to infection. The liver can be tested by measuring the level of enzymes in the blood. These levels are abnormal when there is infection or inflammation (hepatitis) or the liver is unable to perform effectively.

Urine

Simple in-office urine tests are often used to screen for general problems, but they do not provide much information about specific digestive problems. Some naturopaths and nutritionally oriented doctors use a liver detoxification challenge test. Small measured amounts of caffeine, aspirin, and paracetamol are given, and several urine samples are collected at home, along with samples of saliva and blood. These are then sent to the laboratory to determine how efficiently your liver is able to detoxify.

Stool

The stool can provide a wealth of information about digestive processes. One of the simplest tests is for blood in the stool. A small amount of feces is collected and placed in a sample container. Blood that is visible and bright red may well be from hemorrhoids, but the bleeding may not be obvious to the individual. If blood is detected in the test, this points toward conditions such as inflammatory bowel disease, ulcers, and cancer. A positive test result will lead to further testing to establish the cause of the bleeding.

If you have severe diarrhea or unexplained symptoms, your health care practitioner may request a stool sample to test for parasites or bacteria. With more international travel being done and more food being imported, parasitic infections are now fairly common. Evidence of infection may not be present in a stool on a single test, so samples collected over several days may be more useful. Laboratories specializing in parasitology sometimes require a laxative purge to be given before the sample is collected. Parasites like *Giardia* cling to the small intestine wall, but a purge dislodges them sufficiently to be passed into the stool to enable diagnosis.

Comprehensive Digestive Stool Analysis test (CDSA)

The CDSA is a battery of some 20 tests that naturopaths and practitioners of nutritional medicine use, and is often used in the diagnosis of dysbiosis (see p.46 of Conditions). Many conventionally trained doctors are still unfamiliar with these tests, and currently they are available only at specialist centers. The CDSA measures how efficiently the digestive system uses food, and it assesses the activity of the microflora. The CDSA provides evidence on how well an individual digests proteins, fats, and carbohydrates. Protein digestion is inhibited when pancreatic enzyme levels are low, and this may be the cause of flatulence, bloating, and failure to gain weight. If fat absorption is inhibited, it can point to gallbladder problems and deficiencies of the fat-soluble vitamins such as A, D, and E.

If beneficial bacteria are not present in sufficient quantity, or the population of less-welcome visitors increases, a state of dysbiosis exists. This may result in signs and symptoms such as bloating, constipation, diarrhea, fatigue, and flatulence. One of the main offenders is a yeast known as *Candida albicans*. The CDSA indicates the quantities of the specific intestinal flora, and this can be used as the basis for appropriate supplementation or the prescription of antimicrobials.

The CDSA also measures the levels of butyrate produced by the fermentation process in the bowel. This is the major source of energy to the inner wall of the bowel, and low levels of butyrate indicate that the cells are in a state of semi-starvation and not properly nourished.

Intestinal permeability

The intestinal permeability test is used by naturopaths and practitioners of nutritional medicine and is only available at specialist laboratories. A healthy intestinal tract provides an effective barrier against partially digested proteins, toxins, and bacteria entering the bloodstream. If the intestinal tract becomes too permeable and these substances pass into the blood, the body may mount an immunological response, leading to various conditions, from allergy to autoimmune arthritis.

The intestinal permeability test involves drinking a solution containing two harmless compounds, lactulose, which has very large molecules, and mannitol, which has very small molecules. These substances should pass through the system undigested. The quantity found in the urine after the solution is administered indicates how permeable the gut barrier is to molecules of a particular size. The test is used to diagnose leaky gut syndrome (see p.48 of Conditions) and can be retaken to gauge how well the person is responding to therapy.

X-rays

X-rays have long been used to identify problems in the upper and lower digestive tract. Following an overnight fast and before the X-ray of the gut is taken, barium solution is swallowed. This metallic alkaline chemical temporarily coats the lining of the digestive tract, so the lining shows up more clearly on X-ray. The method is useful for diagnosing ulcers, tumors, and strictures of the esophagus. The barium may also be given as an enema when the bowel is the site of investigation. The bowel must be empty when the X-ray is taken. Sometimes an enema is given before the barium is introduced to help empty the colon. As the barium fills the bowel, the radiologist may ask you to turn and hold different positions, to provide the clearest X-rays.

Computed Tomography (CT) Scan

CT scanning combines X-ray images with computer technology to produce three-dimensional images of the internal structures of the body. This method is effective for diagnosing tumors, abscesses, and any other masses deep inside the body. The images can show abnormalities in the liver, gallbladder, and pancreas.

CT scans are taken with the patient lying on a table that slides into a round scanning machine. The procedure is painless and takes from $1/2$ to $1 1/2$ hours. The scanner rotates around the body to take X-rays from various angles. The X-rays are then combined within the computer to produce cross-sectional images of the deep structures of the body.

Magnetic resonance imaging (MRI)

Like the CT scanner, an MRI takes images from different angles, and a computer generates a cross-section of the internal structures of the body; however, there is

This colored X-ray shows the large intestine after a barium enema, a suspension of barium sulphate (which is opaque to x-rays) infused into the rectum.

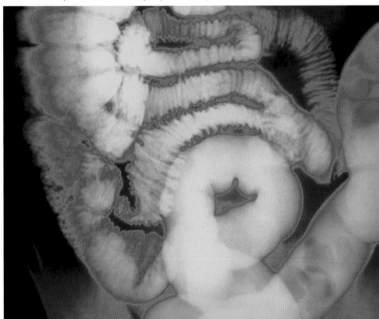

no radiation exposure. Some of the newer MRI scanners are open and do not require the patient to lie in a closed chamber, but the patient must remain still to generate clear images. This makes MRIs less useful for the gastrointestinal tract, in which the peristaltic wave creates ongoing movement, but they are very useful for the liver where they provide the clearest possible images.

Ultrasound

Using high-frequency sound waves and computer technology, images of the internal structures of the body are generated without radiation. A handheld device is placed over the area of the body and sound waves are sent out and reflected back. The computer then reads these signals and displays a two-dimensional image. Ultrasound is often used to examine abdominal organs, such as the liver, gallbladder, and pancreas. It shows whether there are tumors in the organs or gallstones. The whole procedure is completely painless and takes only about $1/2$ hour.

Endoscopy and colonoscopy

An endoscopy is an examination with an endoscope, which is a thin, lighted fiberoptic tube with a tiny camera on the end. The patient is lightly sedated, and the doctor places the endoscope in the patient's mouth; then it is swallowed and goes down the throat to the stomach and duodenum. This allows the doctor to see the lining of the esophagus, stomach, and duodenum. The doctor can use the endoscope to take pictures of any ulcers or remove a tiny piece of tissue (biopsy) to view under a microscope. Sometimes an ultrasound device will be attached to the endoscope to provide additional information (endoscopic ultrasound).

A similar procedure, called a colonoscopy, can be used to gain information about the colon. A laxative or enema may be given before the procedure to ensure the bowel is empty. A full colonoscopy provides information about the whole colon, but a shorter sigmoidoscope only gives information about the lower third of the bowel, where most bowel diseases occur. Sometimes a simpler, quicker procedure can be carried out using a proctoscope, which is an instrument about 4 in (10 cm) long that examines the lowest part of the rectum and anus. Although none of these procedures are very dignified and may be somewhat uncomfortable, they should not be painful.

The acid test

Acid levels in the stomach can be assessed by using an endoscope to draw out a sample of digestive juices for measurement. Sometimes the acid-stimulating hormone gastrin is given and the response measured. These procedures are most commonly used to detect hyperacidity and its relationship to ulcers. Another method to measure stomach acidity is to use a radio transmitter capsule, which sends radio signals to a receiver that records the readings. This capsule is swallowed and provides readings of the acid levels in the upper digestive tract. The capsule may be connected to a thin cord to control how far it goes down the digestive tract and to allow it to be withdrawn, or it may be disposable, in which case it would not need to be recovered after it has passed through the digestive tract.

Allergy and immunity

Food allergies are often suspected as a cause of gastrointestinal symptoms, but it may be quite difficult to discover which foods are the culprits. An elimination diet followed by an oral food challenge may produce the most convincing evidence that certain foods lead to symptoms, but the regimen is difficult and the results can be confusing. This is especially so when there are delayed reactions to foods and more than one food has been introduced at a time. Laboratory tests can provide useful supportive evidence and can be used to focus the elimination regimen on specific foods.

Classic allergy tests use a series of skin pricks or scratches impregnated with potential allergens, and then the skin reaction is evaluated for allergic responses. This method only picks up the immediate IgE immune response, but because these account for only about 10–15 percent of adverse reactions to food, their use is limited.

Tests for IgG may be used to detect delayed allergic reactions to foods. The method is not widely available and tends to be used by practitioners of nutritional medicine. The link between raised IgG levels and clinical symptoms is unproven. A small sample of blood is taken and a fraction of the blood is put in contact with a series of 30–150 potential allergens, depending on the profile requested. Using sensitive measuring equipment, the fraction of blood is then examined for the presence of IgG antibodies. If the levels are raised, this indicates that the body has developed an immune response to the food.

Secretory immunoglobulin A testing

The body's first immune defense against bacteria, parasites, toxins, and viruses in the digestive tract is secretory IgA. This antibody is found in the saliva and the secretions from the mucous membranes of the entire digestive tract. If levels of this antibody are low, the immunity against foreign substances may be compromised. The test requires a sample of saliva or stool to evaluate the status of the mucosal immunity. These tests are generally performed by a nutritionist.

Gluten intolerance

Antibody testing can be used to diagnose specific conditions. IgA testing for antigliadin antibody is used as the first step in diagnosing celiac disease. Gliadin is the part of gluten to which people have a toxic reaction. If this test is positive and the symptoms suggest celiac disease, a small tissue sample (biopsy) may be taken with an endoscope to confirm the diagnosis.

Candida albicans

Tests for *Candida albicans* are not routinely used by conventional medical practitioners, but some naturopaths and nutritionally oriented doctors find them useful. The body's immune response to *Candida* can be established by IgG testing. A high IgG level suggests that the body has had an ongoing immune response to the yeast. The presence of IgM antibodies reflects a more current response by the immune system to candida. Stool cultures provide some quantitative evaluation of the proliferation of *Candida* in the gut. The results of all these tests need to be interpreted cautiously. By themselves, positive antibody or culture test results don't accurately reflect whether someone has candidiasis. A detailed medical history and diagnostic questionnaire can help establish whether candiasis is present and possibly contributing to current health problems.

Lactose intolerance

As discussed in the section on food intolerance, some adverse reactions to food cannot be classed as allergies because they do not evoke the characteristic immune response. Some people have an inability to digest the lactose in milk products (cheese may be tolerated because the milk has been through a process of fermentation). An

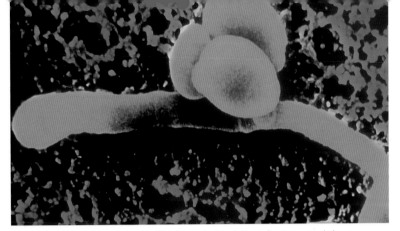
Candida albicans *is the yeastlike fungi behind the infection candidiasis.*

excess of hydrogen occurs when the bacteria in the colon ferment the undigested lactose and leads to symptoms of bloating and diarrhea. Lactose intolerance is tested for by measuring the breath for hydrogen excreted after drinking milk.

Vega and other electroacupuncture testing

Vega and other electroacupuncture testing use a galvanometer to measure the skin's electrical resistance at designated acupuncture points. The patient holds a negative electrode in one hand and the positive electrode is pressed on selected acupuncture points, while the suspected food in a glass ampule is placed in a tray connected into the circuit. Changes in the galvanometer readings indicate sensitivity. However, because a credible explanation on the test's mode of operation is lacking, it must be considered subjective and should not be relied upon, until research is able to demonstrate its reliability and validity.

Applied kinesiology

In applied kinesiology, certain muscles are tested for strength by having the person resist moving a limb, and then placing a sample of the suspect foods in the patient's mouth or on the patient's skin. The muscles are then retested. Muscle weakness as perceived by the examiner is considered to be a positive test result. Several good quality studies have failed to demonstrate that the test results of applied kinesiology can be reliably reproduced. Unless it can be demonstrated that the method is repeatable and valid, applied kinesiology should not be relied upon because the implications for the patient may be unnecessary and dangerous.

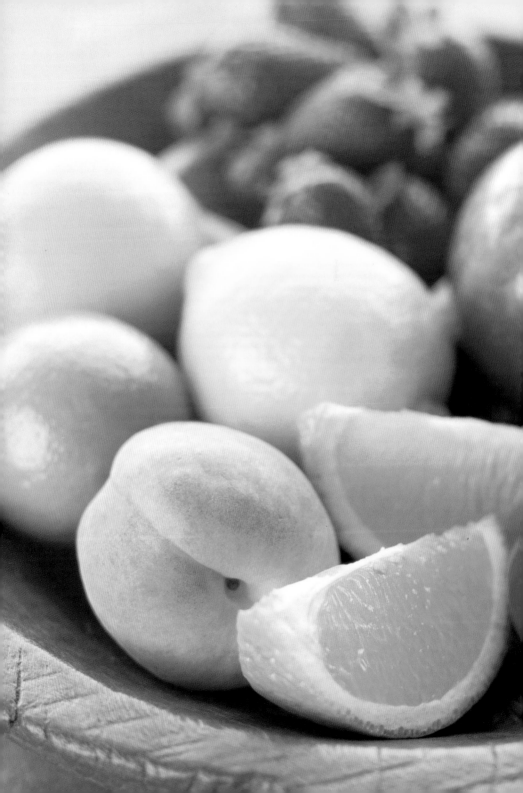

options
for
health

The following section discusses a range of lifestyle and dietary modifications to promote better digestion and help with the symptoms of digestive disease. Advice is easy to give but not necessarily so easy to follow. There are many reasons for this. Force of habit makes all change difficult. Another reason is not understanding why or how to bring about changes and incorporate them into daily life. This section offers lots of practical advice to get you started, and once you feel the benefits you should find it easier not to relapse into old habits.

lifestyle
changes

Sometimes when many small things contribute to deteriorating health, people do not know where to start. First aim to make small changes that seem realistic. If you feel the benefit of the changes and begin to break the inertia of the old habits, then this becomes a positive reinforcement for further changes. Having a goal that you want to achieve is also a stimulus for change. Therefore, try to plan the steps you will take to reach your goal and the modifications you will make if some aspect proves to be unachievable.

Breaking bad habits is hard, even when one knows the dangers of letting them continue. Most smokers smoke in spite of knowing that it damages the lungs and cause cancer. People put off changing their habits for another day and risk their health. Some hope and vaguely plan that they will manage to give up before they become ill, others feel that their life would not be worth living without the luxury of their habit.

Improving your digestion sometimes requires that you look beyond diet and specific treatments. Many digestive conditions are aggravated—if not caused—by stress and lifestyle factors. Although specific treatments can certainly be important, the key to improvement is often a question of achieving balance in eating, sleeping, exercising, and effectively managing the stresses of modern living. The term *stress* is vague, because many kinds of stress exist. There are physical stresses and strains on the body as well as psychological ones. If the body's chemistry is not functioning correctly, this can also cause stress on the body and mind.

Although it is beyond the scope of this book to discuss in detail how each of these important areas of influence can enhance or undermine your health, it is worth giving a name to some of them. The research showing the effect of social support in recovering from cancer and other serious diseases is very convincing. The influence on health of such areas as leisure, play, and creativity has not been as extensively researched but is likely to be no less important. The circle diagram below names some of these areas of life. Although these may not reflect exactly your own set of priorities, they should give you an idea of how to view the interrelated aspects of life and allow you to consider the areas you think are important. To try and get a sense of how these areas may be influencing your well-being, you could score your level of satisfaction in the areas that have been identified (or create your own if these do not reflect your own priorities). Zero is very dissatisfied, and ten is highly satisfied. If your scores are in the upper numbers, these areas are likely to be having a positive influence on your health. If the scores

EVALUATE YOUR LIFESTYLE IN THESE AREAS

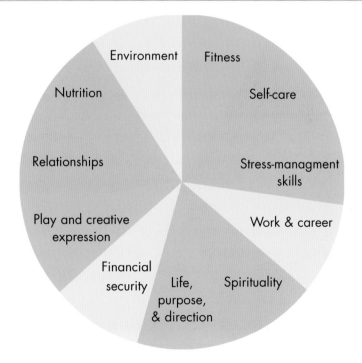

are at the lower end, it may mean that your well-being and health are being compromised. It may not be practicable to make dramatic changes in each area, but even identifying difficult areas can make you more alert to opportunities for improvement. Taking responsibility for your own well-being can be a positive step in itself, and often is the first and most important step to improved health.

What to eat

The principles of good diet are really quite simple. Eat a wide variety of fresh natural foods, looking for organic produce where possible. The emphasis should be on plant-based foods with plenty of vegetables, fruit, and foods made from whole grains and dried beans and legumes. These supply carbohydrate, protein, fiber, and fats as well as beneficial vitamins, minerals, and phytochemicals (compounds within plants that exert a beneficial effect).

Fiber

Plant foods are an excellent source of fiber. Getting enough fiber helps many common conditions related to colon function, including constipation, hemorrhoids, and diverticulosis; protects you from some forms of cancer; and significantly reduces your risk of heart disease, diabetes, and obesity.

There are two kinds of fiber—insoluble and soluble. Insoluble fiber from wheat, rice, and maize increases the stool bulk. The increased bulk speeds up the transit time of feces and reduces pressure in your bowel. Reduced pressure helps prevent diverticular disease. When people increase their fiber intake, it is not uncommon to experience a temporary increase in flatulence. This should pass in a couple of weeks as the body gets used to the change in diet. People with IBS who are not able to tolerate taking insoluble fiber should rely on soluble sources of fiber, which is found in most fruit, vegetables, legumes, and oats.

Unless adequate fluids are taken with fiber, it can be constipating. Soluble fiber absorbs up to fifteen times its own weight in water, which helps to soften the stool. Another benefit is that when soluble fiber comes in contact with bile acids, it binds with them and carries them out of the body. Bile acids are rich in cholesterol and much of it is normally reabsorbed, unless it becomes bound with soluble fiber and is carried out of the body.

Adequate fiber intake is also important for maintaining a healthy balance of microflora in the gut. An additional benefit of fiber-rich foods is that they slow the rate of absorption of carbohydrates. This results in a more gradual release of sugar into the blood, which is beneficial for disorders such as diabetes and reactive hypoglycemia. The bulk within fiber foods makes you feel full and therefore less likely to overeat.

ENERGY REQUIREMENT

MALES
The amount of daily energy that a man needs varies according to age and lifestyle. Average requirements are listed below, although there is much variation within each group.

FEMALES
The amount of energy that a woman needs for daily life is generally lower than that of a man. However, extra calories are needed during pregnancy and breast-feeding.

Age	Kcal per day	Age	Kcal per day
0–3 months	545	0–3 months	515
4–6 months	690	4–6 months	645
7–9 months	825	7–9 months	765
10–12 months	920	10–12 months	865
1–3 years	1,230	1–3 years	1,165
4–6 years	1,715	4–6 years	1,545
7–10 years	1,970	7–10 years	1,740
11–14 years	2,220	11–14 years	1,845
15–18 years	2,755	15–18 years	2,110
19–50 years	2,550	19–50 years	1,940
51–59 years	2,550	51–59 years	1,900
60–64 years	2,380	60–64 years	1,900
65–74 years	2,330	65–74 years	1,900
75+ years	2,100	75+ years	1,810

Additional Requrements for Women	Kcal per day
Pregnancy (third trimester)	+200
Breast-feeding	+450 to 480

Energy

The energy requirements for an individual vary greatly and are determined by age, activity level, and metabolic rate. Special periods—such as growth, pregnancy, and breast-feeding—require more energy. The basic unit of energy is called a calorie (Kcal). The more you do, the more calories you burn, although about 70 percent of your total energy expenditure goes to maintaining basic functions such as breathing, circulation, and nervous system activity. Although subject to wide variations, an adult man requires about 2,500 Kcal per day to maintain normal weight and an adult woman requires about 2,000 Kcal; the amount required decreases as the person gets older, especially so if the person becomes sedentary. Energy taken in excess of these requirements leads to the calories being stored as fat and over a period of time to obesity. To lose weight, the body must use more calories than it takes in.

To estimate whether you are a healthy weight, you can use a formula called the Body Mass Index (BMI). The BMI is your weight in kilograms divided by the square of your height in meters. It is an estimate of your total body fat. People with a BMI of between 25 and 29.9 kilograms per meter squared (kg/m^2) are overweight, those with a BMI of 30–39.9kg/m^2 are obese, and those with a BMI of 40kg/m^2 or more are severely obese. Use the chart by locating your height on the left-hand column and following it across till your locate your weight. Then you can use the formula described above to work out your BMI.

The sources of energy for the body come from carbohydrates, proteins, and fats. The energy value of a food depends on the relative proportion of these components. Weight-for-weight fat contains about twice the amount of calories compared to a carbohydrate or protein, although fat is not the ideal primary source of energy.

Carbohydrates

Complex carbohydrates should be the main source of energy for the body. These come from grains such as cereals, rice, bread, and pasta, as well as from starchy vegetables such as potato, butternut squash, yams, corn, and parsnip. As well as providing the body with slow-burn energy, they are an important source of many vitamins, minerals, and fiber. Some people with digestive disorders have difficulty

WHAT SHOULD YOU WEIGH?

To find out whether you are a healthy weight for your height, first find your weight on the left side of the chart below. Then run your finger across to your height and see in which of the three sections you fall.

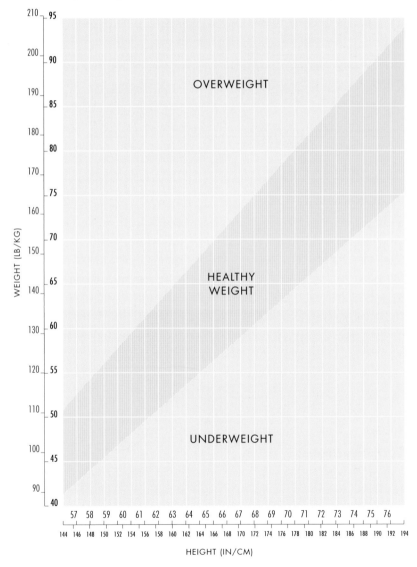

WEIGHT (LB/KG)

OVERWEIGHT

HEALTHY WEIGHT

UNDERWEIGHT

HEIGHT (IN/CM)

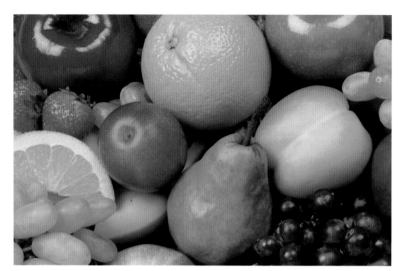

Most fruit have a low or medium glycemic index, and are an important component of a healthy diet.

tolerating wheat products and other gluten-containing grains, such as barley, rye, and possibly oats. Some of the products made from wheat include pasta, couscous, cracked wheat, bulghur, and wheat bran. Other carbohydrates that people with a wheat intolerance may be able to tolerate include rice, starchy vegetables such as potato, parsnip, and corn products, including corn on the cob, cornmeal, polenta, and popped corn. Buckwheat, quinoa, and amaranth are grainlike seeds that can provide useful additions to carbohydrate intake. Select whole grains such as brown rice or whole-grain pasta because these unrefined products supply the body with important nutrients such as minerals and fiber.

Sugars Sugars provide immediate energy for the body. Glucose is the main fuel that the cells of the body use and the blood sugar levels must be maintained for the body to function effectively. Blood sugar levels are regulated by insulin, a hormone secreted by the pancreas, that must be kept within a narrow limit. When the body has a plentiful supply of sugar the liver and muscles store what the body does not need for immediate use as glycogen. If the reserves of glycogen are full any excess sugar eaten is stored as fat.

THE GLYCEMIC INDEX

Cause a rapid rise in the blood sugar level (foods with a high glycemic index)

Cereals
White bread
Whole-grain/wheat bread
White rice
Brown rice
Rye crispbread
Plain crackers

Breakfast cereals
Cornflakes
All frosted cereals
Muesli
Shredded Wheat
Weetabix

Biscuits and Confectionery
Boiled sweets
Most sweet chocolate bars
Toffee
Fudge
Nougat

Vegetables
Carrots
Parsnips
Sweet corn
Broad beans
Potatoes (boiled, baked, or instant)

Fruit
Raisins
Bananas

Cause a moderate rise in the blood sugar level (foods with a moderate glycemic index)

Cereals
Pasta
Noodles
Oats

Breakfast cereals
Porridge
Bran
Oat bran

Biscuits and confectionery
Oat cakes
Plain/sweet biscuits (rich tea, etc)
Sponge cake

Vegetables
Sweet potatoes
Yams

Fruit
Grapes
Oranges

Causes a slow rise in the blood sugar level (foods with a low glycemic index)

Vegetables
Butter beans
Baked beans
Chickpeas
Haricot beans
Lentils
Kidney beans
Soybeans
Peanuts

Fruit
Apples
Cherries
Dates
Figs
Grapefruit
Peaches
Pears
Plums

Dairy products
Milk (whole and skimmed)
Yogurt (plain and fruit)
Ice cream

Sugars
Fructose

The glycemic index (GI) of a food measures the rate at which it raises blood sugar levels. For many years it had been assumed that all complex carbohydrates were broken down slowly into simple sugars, leading to a gradual increase in the blood sugar level, and that simple sugars rapidly increase the blood sugar level. Simple sugars are glucose, sucrose (table sugar), fructose (in fruit), and galactose (milk sugar). However, this assumption is an oversimplification, and studies over the last decade measuring the effects of different foods on blood sugar levels have shown that some foods rich in complex carbohydrates (such as bread, rice, and potatoes) can also rapidly increase the blood sugar levels. This is because these foods contain a form of the starch that the body rapidly digests and absorbs. The type of starch, particle size, maturation of a fruit or vegetable, cooking time, and many other factors affect the glycemic index. Some simple sugars, such as fructose (which is found in fruit and honey), have a relatively low glycemic index. This does not mean that you should avoid foods with a high GI altogether but instead you should combine low and high GI foods with an emphasis on plant foods that provide a low GI for a balanced diet.

Vegetables and fruit Most vegetables and fruit are naturally low in calories and almost fat-free, except for avocados and olives, which contain high-quality fatty acids. Vegetables provide a rich source of vitamins, minerals, fiber, and phytochemicals, such as the antioxidant carotenes. They are the richest source of antioxidants—the compounds that destroy disease-producing free radicals. Many vegetables can be enjoyed in their fresh raw form, however, if cooked, it is important not to overcook them because this leads to loss of nutrients as well as flavor.

Proteins

Proteins are made up from building blocks called amino acids, which are necessary to build and repair all the tissues of the body. The body can manufacture some amino acids, but eight essential ones must be obtained from the diet. These are best obtained by eating various protein-rich foods. Although recommended daily requirements vary due to factors such as age, sex, and body size, most people need 35–45 gm per day. This may be calculated as 0.6–0.8 gm per kg body mass per day. Many people living in the developed world eat far in excess of this amount and

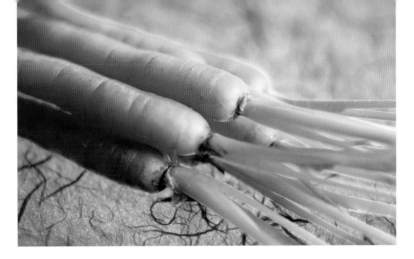

Vegetables such as carrots are low in calories, contain virtually no fat, and are high in many essential vitamins, minerals, and antioxidants. Eaten raw, they are a nutritious snack food.

create an unnecessary burden upon the body's eliminative systems. A simple way to reduce this excessive intake is to increase the amount of plant food you eat.

Meat, fish, poultry Meat, fish and poultry provide complete proteins—that is, they contain all the essential amino acids the body requires. The problem with meat is that even lean cuts contain fat and cholesterol. You should always choose low-fat cuts and remove the skin from poultry before eating. Use these foods as side dishes rather than the main part of a meal. The exception is cold-water fish such as salmon, mackerel, cod, and halibut, which all contain omega-3 fatty acids. The value of these fatty acids is that they reduce the risk of diseases such as heart disease, stroke, autoimmune diseases such as inflammatory bowel disease and rheumatoid arthritis, eczema, and allergies.

Dairy and eggs As well as providing an excellent balance of amino acids, eggs and dairy foods such as milk, cheese, and yogurt are good sources of calcium and of vitamin D, which helps the body absorb calcium. Because dairy foods are high in saturated fats and cholesterol, you should limit consumption of these foods. Eggs do not increase the level of blood cholesterol and they are an excellent source of protein. Because the diet of the chickens influences the balance of essential fatty acids in the eggs, choose free-range and organic eggs where possible.

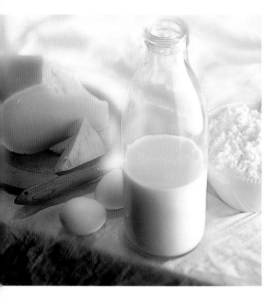

Dairy foods are a good source of calcium, but they are also high in saturated fats and cholesterol.

Beans, legumes, and cereals
Certain plant foods are rich in complete protein, such as soybeans and the soy products soy milk, tofu, and tempeh. Cereals and dried beans and legumes, such as dried peas and lentils, are good sources of amino acids, but you should include a variety of these foods in your daily diet to ensure that you are obtaining all the essential amino acids the body requires.

Nuts and seeds As well as providing an excellent source of protein, nuts are a rich source of essential fatty acids. Although the body cannot produce essential fatty acids, it is important not to eat nuts excessively because of their high calorie content. A handful of almonds or sunflower seeds can make a good protein-rich snack. Pine nuts, cashews, and almonds can be added to various vegetable and grain dishes for extra flavor and protein. Avoid using peanut butter excessively because it has a high fat content, and peanuts often contain a low level of aflatoxin, a mold known to cause cancer when taken in high quantities.

Fats

As well as being the most concentrated source of energy, the fats in your diet supply essential fatty acids (EFAs) and the fat-soluble vitamins A, D, E, and K. The body needs the fatty acids linoleic acid and linolenic acid, cannot manufacture them, and cannot survive without them. These substances are important components of nerve cells, cellular membranes and hormone-like substances called prostaglandins. They are also important in the transport, breakdown, and excretion of cholesterol. The amount and type of fatty acids you eat influences the way your body handles them. The richest sources of EFAs are flaxseed oil, avocados, olives, seeds, nuts, and cold-water fish.

Saturated fats are those that tend to be solid at room temperature. The main source of these in the diet comes from animal fats such as butter and the fat within meats. Vegetable fats and fish oils, which are liquid at room temperature are described as unsaturated fats. A high saturated fat diet is linked to heart disease and stroke as well as various cancers, such as colorectal and breast cancer. Your total fat intake should be kept well below 30 percent of your total calorie intake, with a much higher proportion of unsaturated fats compared to saturated fats. Unfortunately, few vegetable oils are healthy because of the way they are processed and refined. The heat used to process most oils changes their chemical structure from the beneficial *cis* form to the more harmful *trans* form.

Most people in the USA and UK eat more total fat and saturated fat than recommended. There are various ways to correct this imbalance. Choose lower fat dairy products or use less of the full-fat variety. Use less fat in cooking and fewer spreads, such as butter or margarine. Grill and bake rather than frying or roasting. Choose lower-fat cuts of meat and remove the skin from poultry. Replace saturated fats with ones richer in monounsaturated fatty acids (olive oil or rapeseed oil) and polyunsaturated fatty acids (cold-pressed sunflower or corn oil). Margarine, even if it is polyunsaturated, is best avoided.

To make a vegetable oil that is to be solid at room temperature, manufacturers use a process called hydrogenation, which alters the chemical structure of the fatty acid from the beneficial *cis* form to the harmful *trans* form. These transfatty acids block the normal function of cis-fatty acids and have been associated with hardening of the arteries (atherosclerosis) and heart disease as well as inflammatory conditions such as arthritis. Nonhydrogenated margarines may be available at health food stores, or you can simply use small quantities of butter—or, even better, use a little olive oil.

Some dietary fats are visible (such as butter, cooking oils, and the fat on meat), whereas others are invisible (such as those in cakes, biscuits, and prepared foods), so if you are not careful, your fat intake can increase dramatically. One of the main reasons fats are used is that they improve the taste of many foods and because they take time to pass through the stomach, they provide a satisfying feeling of fullness. It is important to be aware how much and what kind of fat you are eating. Look carefully at the packaging of prepared foods to evaluate the hidden fat content.

Serving size

Serving size is very important in maintaining good health. It is easy to be deceived about your intake of food. You may have one piece of cake but the size of the slice can vary enormously. If you eat a larger portion, count it as more than one serving. A large plate of pasta for lunch is more likely to be two or three servings than one.

The US Department of Agriculture has produced a pyramid that provides a visual representation of the recommended portions for the different food groups. They are divided into the following food groups.

Grains sit at the base of the pyramid, and the recommended daily intake is a minimum of 6–11 servings. These should come predominantly from whole grains and whole-grain bread. Although this sounds like a lot, you will be surprised at how they add up in a day. Equivalent to one serving is 1 slice of bread, 1 oz (28 gms) of ready-to-eat cereal, or $^1/_2$ cup of cooked cereal, rice, or pasta.

Fruit and vegetables are at the next level of the pyramid, and you should have a minimum of 5 servings, with up to 9 daily. You can choose freely whether on any day to have more fruit or vegetables, but the overall minimum should be five servings. A serving is equivalent to 1 cup of raw leafy vegetables; $^1/_2$ cup of other fruits and vegetables, cooked or chopped raw; or $^3/_4$ cup of fruit or vegetable juice.

Protein-rich foods are at the next level of the pyramid. For meat, poultry, fish, dried beans, eggs, and nuts, 2–3 servings are the minimum recommended intake. A serving is equivalent to 2–3 oz (50–75 gm) of cooked lean meat, poultry, or fish; 1 cup of cooked dry beans such as lentils; or $^1/_2$ cup of nuts.

For eggs and dairy foods—which include milk, yogurt, and cheese—2–3 servings is the recommended minimum. A serving is equivalent to 1 cup of milk or yogurt, $1^1/_2$ oz (40 g) of natural cheese, or two eggs.

It is important to maintain the proportion of protein-rich foods such as meat and dairy foods to carbohydrate, fruit, and vegetables, which should predominate. If you have an intolerance to dairy foods or eggs, then you can obtain nutrients from other foods rich in protein and calcium, such as soybeans, nuts, and cold-water fish.

Use fats, oils, and sweets sparingly. The intake again needs to be proportional to the rest of the food groups in the pyramid. Your intake of polyunsaturated fats should be equal to or greater than your intake of saturated fats.

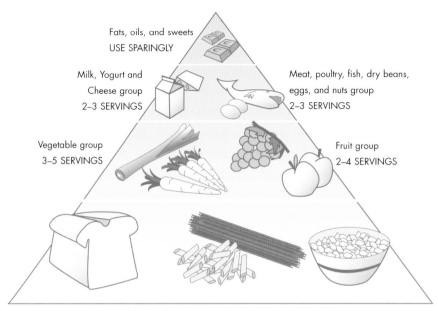

Fats, oils, and sweets
USE SPARINGLY

Milk, Yogurt and
Cheese group
2–3 SERVINGS

Meat, poultry, fish, dry beans,
eggs, and nuts group
2–3 SERVINGS

Vegetable group
3–5 SERVINGS

Fruit group
2–4 SERVINGS

Bread, cereal, rice, & pasta group   6–11 SERVINGS

FOOD PYRAMID – a guide to daily food choices

How many calories do you need?

Whereas the proportion between the food groups should be maintained, the number of servings that are right for you depends on how many calories you need, which in turn depends on your age, sex, size, and activity level. The table on p.88 provides an approximate guide, based on a lower, moderate, and higher calorie intake. As a guide, the lower calorie intake of 1,600 will maintain the weight of many sedentary women and some older adults. The moderate calorie intake of 2,200 is appropriate for most children, teenage girls, active women, and many sedentary men (this need may increase to some extent for women who are pregnant or breast-feeding). The higher intake of 2,800 calories is suitable for teenage boys, many active men, and some very active women.

What to avoid

To maintain good health and improve your digestion, you should limit or avoid certain things altogether. The first among these is best described as excess. Avoid eating excess food as well as specific substances like fats, salt, sugar, and alcohol. Although not a food, tobacco in any form is positively harmful to digestion and health in general. Many digestive problems can be avoided if this first rule is maintained. Now look at each in turn.

Fat and cholesterol The body needs cholesterol and manufactures 95 percent itself, which it uses to make steroid hormones and maintain the integrity of cellular membranes. Cholesterol is also a component of the bile excreted by the liver. However, the more saturated fat in your diet, the higher your blood cholesterol level becomes. In particular, saturated fats lead to an increase in low-density lipoproteins (LDL). It is this "bad" LDL cholesterol that is then deposited in the arteries making them narrower (atherosclerosis). This can lead to a heart attack if the arteries supplying the heart become blocked, or to a stroke if the blood flow to a part of the brain is occluded. An excessive intake of cholesterol may also lead to gallstone formation. Normally bile coming from the liver contains enough bile salts and lecithin to keep the cholesterol dissolved. Cholesterol, however, is not easily soluble and if the bile has more cholesterol than can be dissolved, the excess cholesterol can form into crystals and fuse into stones within the gallbladder. The

FOOD GROUPS AND CALORIE INTAKE	Lower 1,600 Kcal	Moderate 2,200 Kcal	Higher 2,800 Kcal
Grain group servings	6	9	11
Vegetable group servings	3	4	5
Fruit group servings	2	3	4
Milk group servings	2–3	2–3	2–3
Meat group	2–3	2–3	2–3
Simple sugars (table, honey, dried fruits)	6	12	18
Total fat (grams)	53	73	93

causes are complex and influenced by obesity and a genetic predisposition, but a low fat—rather than no-fat—diet predominantly coming from unsaturated fats (especially olive oil) is recommended. Olive oil is rich in high-density lipoproteins. This "good" form of lipoprotein picks up and removes cholesterol from the blood and takes it to the liver for elimination.

Salt Table salt is the common name for sodium chloride, a mixture that is 40 percent sodium and 60 percent chloride. The recommended limit for sodium intake is about 2,400 mg per day (about 1 1/4 teaspoons of table salt), but many people get much more than this, even without adding salt at the table. Processed foods, including canned foods, cured meats, frozen dinners, and commercially baked goods, such as cookies and pastries, contain the most sodium. Bread and cheese are also typically high in sodium.

Some people are particularly sodium sensitive, and high sodium intake leads to high blood pressure, which is a risk factor for stroke, heart disease, and kidney failure. The general recommendation for healthy people without high blood pressure is 2,400 mg daily. The typical American or British diet contains 4,000–6,000 mg per day. If you have high blood pressure, reducing sodium to 2,400–3,000 mg a day would make a very good start. To get less than 2,000 mg a day, you need to check labels carefully and seek out special low-sodium foods.

Sugar Refined simple sugars, which include, sucrose (table sugar), glucose, fructose, and galactose (the sugar from milk) are rich in calories but contribute little else to the diet, which is why they are sometimes called empty calories. It is good advice to avoid excessive intake of these substances. Unfortunately not only do these sweeteners help pile on the pounds, excessive intake of them leads to disturbances of blood sugar metabolism. How quickly the sugar gets into the bloodstream is measured by the glycemic index. A diet with a high glycemic load increases the risk of diabetes, raises the "bad" LDL cholesterol levels, and promotes faster weight gain and higher body-fat levels. A diet high in refined sugars and carbohydrates that are quickly absorbed into the bloodstream (such as bread, white rice, and potatoes) increases the glycemic load very quickly. Refined sugar has also been shown to have a depressive effect on the immune system by inhibiting the

WATCHING YOUR SODIUM LEVELS

To keep within the recommended healthy range:
- choose fresh fruits and vegetables as often as possible
- look for sodium-free varieties of frozen and canned vegetables, if you use them
- use salt-free seasonings (such as herbs, spices, and vinegar) in cooking and at the table
- avoid adding salt when cooking pasta, rice, or vegetables
- choose fewer salty snacks such as salted nuts, popcorn, chips, pretzels, and crackers
- read food labels for sodium content.

ability of the white blood cells (neutrophils) to engulf and destroy bacteria. This is in addition to the well-known effects that sugar has on increasing dental caries.

Carbonated drinks Fizzy drinks introduce extra gas into the digestive system and cause bloating and wind in the upper digestive tract. This may lead to discomfort in the abdomen or even chest pain. Plain water and juices are better options.

Alcohol Excessive and continuous use of alcohol is very damaging to the digestive tract. It is a major cause of gastritis, ulcers, cirrhosis, and liver damage as well as inflammation throughout the digestive tract. Pancreatitis and disturbance of the blood sugar regulating mechanism are induced by long-term heavy drinking.

There is evidence that one or two servings of alcohol a day has a protective effect on the heart (due to the apparent antioxidant effect of flavinoids in wine, particularly red), but this benefit needs to be balanced against the irritant effect of alcohol on the gut. A serving is equivalent to a 5 fl oz (150 ml) glass of wine, a pint of beer, or a 5 fl oz (150 ml) measure of spirits. If you have digestive problems, you are probably better off avoiding alcohol altogether or at least cutting down dramatically. Consider using exercise (a workout, run, or yoga) or relaxation (perhaps a soak in the bath) to serve as a transition from the daytime and work to the relaxation of the evening.

Tobacco The ill effects of tobacco are many. Cigarettes contain over 400 toxic substances. The most damaging is tar, which can cause lung cancer. Carbon monoxide and nicotine can contribute to cardiovascular disease, and the particulate matter and gases can cause chronic obstructive pulmonary disease. Nicotine is an irritant that inflames the lining of the stomach. Smoking is a major risk factor for ulcers, with the rate of healing being slower and the rate of relapse being higher.

Smokers dramatically increase their risk of cancer. Cancers of the mouth, throat, and lung hardly ever affect nonsmokers. Smokers double their risk of stomach cancer. Of all cases of lung cancer, 85 percent are related to smoking and a smoker is 12 times more likely to develop lung cancer than a nonsmoker. If a smoker quits, it takes about 15 years before their risk of getting lung cancer is the same as a nonsmoker.

Smoker's lung (chronic obstructive pulmonary disease) typically starts when a person is 35–45 years of age. At that age, lung function starts to decline even in nonsmokers, and in susceptible smokers, the rate of decline in lung function can be three times the usual rate. As lung function declines, breathlessness on exertion starts. At first, smoker's lung consists of a cough and sputum, which are the signs of bronchitis. As the condition progresses, the person feels short of breath climbing stairs, walking up a slope, or even upon walking. Severe short-term problems will usually require several periods of hospital care. The final stage is a very distressing death due to slow and relentlessly progressive breathlessness. Too many people die every year from this disease which, in 80 percent of cases, is caused by smoking. Giving up smoking at any stage reduces the rate of decline, but stopping the habit is for many people an ongoing struggle. The key starting point is to set a date and make a commitment to stick to it. There are various supportive measures such as nicotine patches, acupuncture, hypnosis, and behavior modification therapies. Without the basic level of commitment, these measures are doomed to failure, but if the motivation is in place, they may offer support to quit the habit.

Relaxing and managing stress

Stress is one of the main triggers that aggravates digestive conditions. Stress sensitizes the gastrointestinal tract. The network of nerve fibers in the gut are

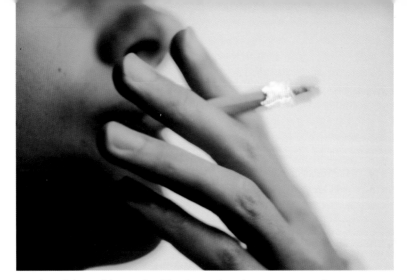

Besides all the well-known health risks, such as lung cancer, smoking is a major risk factor for stomach ulcers.

extensive and make the gut highly responsive to psychological stress. It is not just the nervous system that affects gut activity. Gut function is also regulated by hormones released within the gastrointestinal tract and many other sites in the body. These neurological and chemical transmitters act as an interface between the mind and the body, traveling in both directions—from the mind to the body (psychosomatic) and from the body to the mind (somatopsychic).

When stressed, your body responds as though it is in danger by pumping extra blood into your muscles. This is called the fight-or-flight response, a primitive reaction to enable you to defend yourself against attack or to run away. When the fight-or-flight response is activated, less blood is directed toward the digestive organs to support digestion, the digestive muscles work less, digestive enzymes are secreted in smaller amounts, and the passage of food through the tract slows, leading to heartburn, bloating, and constipation. Sometimes the stress response produces the opposite effects, and food speeds though the digestive tract and causes abdominal pain and diarrhea.

For some people, the gut is a barometer that reflects their worry or anxiety; the gut is a target organ for stress. Whether or not mental and emotional stress causes disease, it can aggravate an existing condition. This can become a vicious circle where the symptoms are made worse by stress, which results in increased mental and emotional stress. Stress affects behavior, and the strategies

THE KEY DIETARY PRINCIPLES
1   Choose a diet rich in a variety of plant-based foods.
2   Eat plenty of fruits and vegetables.
3   Maintain a healthy weight, and be physically active.
4   Drink alcohol only in moderation.
5   Select foods low in fat and sodium.
6   Minimize your intake of sugary foods and drinks.

you use may not always be the most helpful, for example, using alcohol and drugs. Becoming more aware of how your body responds is the first step to bringing about a change. Those same mind-body pathways that create stress can also be used to soothe stress.

The effects of stress may be experienced at different levels. Your body may tell you before your mind does that you are struggling with too much stress. The signs and symptoms include muscle tension, aches and pains, fatigue; and digestive signs and symptoms such as diarrhea, constipation, and indigestion. Mental and emotional symptoms include worry, irritability, mood swings, and poor concentration. Behaviors that point to difficulty managing stress include drug and alcohol overuse, poor eating habits, and especially overeating.

There are many methods to relieve stress, including listening to music or playing music, engaging in gentle exercise such as walking, practicing specific techniques such as yoga or meditation, and receiving a massage. This section describes how you can use relaxation and meditation to relieve stress.

Meditation

The word *meditation* means different things to different people, and there are various forms of it. Often seen as a technique or method to help combat the stresses and strains of modern living, meditation may also be part of a personal development program or spiritual practice. It is all of these things, but meditation is also a naturally occurring state of awareness common to all people at certain moments in their life. This state is so absorbing that the outside world and time itself seem to disappear. For some, these moments come while they are out in the countryside, involved in a sport, or even walking, playing, or listening to music or relaxing in the bath. The common thread to all these activities is a free-flowing state of awareness, being totally in the moment, not dwelling upon the past, or the future, but being fully open to the present.

These naturally occurring states can be cultivated and enhanced by learning more about the meditative state and the various ways of reaching it. When people learn a method of meditation, they are often struck by its simplicity. That does not mean it is always easy, the challenge is in staying focused on the meditation process. Meditation requires the opposite of effort, which is letting go.

Once you acquire the habit of meditation, it gets easier and easier to return to that state. As in a physical sport like golf, a beginner may from time to time hit the ball perfectly, but to play the game with any skill requires regular practice. Everyone falls into spontaneous meditative states from time to time, but if you want to get the benefits that accrue from meditation, you need to practice regularly. Like all forms of exercise, meditation becomes easier with practice. Creating a peaceful area at home where you will not be disturbed will help you establish a daily meditation routine.

Three approaches to meditation Meditation practices can be categorized into three types, according to the essential purpose behind your desire to meditate at any particular time.

1 Mindfulness meditation: In this classic type of meditation, you seek to observe yourself in a passive, relaxed way. You are patient and trusting, letting go and accepting whatever you find, in a nonjudgmental way.

2 Working the will: In this type of meditation, you seek personal development using a combination of meditation and visualization techniques and affirmations—for example, to replace a negative pattern with a good one, to overcome a fear, or to heal a particular part of your body.

3 Inner focus, outer focus: In this type of meditation, you focus inward—either on the internal workings of your body or consciousness—or outward by opening up your mind to the world around.

Preparing to meditate Before embarking on a particular meditation, it is essential to set the scene, both in terms of the environment and the readiness of your mind and body.

1 Make sure you have enough time: If possible set up a regular time of day in which to meditate.

2 Ensure that the space you choose is peaceful and comfortable, and that you will not be interrupted—for example, adjust the lighting and music appropriately.

3 Make sure your body is comfortable: It is better not to meditate on a full stomach or under the influence of alcohol.

4 Do not meditate if you are agitated about something: Exercise first to release pent-up energy from your body.

5 If your mind will not disengage from rational thought, try focusing on an image.

6 Distance yourself from everyday concerns as you walk toward your place of meditation—that is, locate yourself.

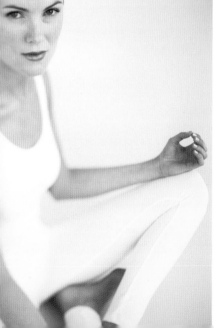

A meditation on being at home in your body The body is the source of all feelings. It is where life experiences are stored. Every day you carry pleasure and joy as well as stress and strain, often without being fully aware of just what you are holding onto. These feelings may become locked

---

The main challenge that meditation offers is to stay focused. But if you perservere with your practice, it is an extremely effective stress-management tool.

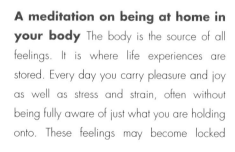

away in our body. Bringing awareness to the feelings in your body is an important form of meditation, helping to ground experience and build confidence in your body and yourself.

Bringing the mind and body together Your mind and body work together as one inseparable, interconnected unit. At times when your mind is spinning with thoughts, you may lose the sense of connection with your own body and then lose touch with the sources of your feelings of pleasure or stress. This meditation can put you back in touch with your feelings and allow you to resolve or come to terms with stressful and difficult feelings and to enjoy and enhance peaceful and pleasurable feelings.

Draw your attention inward Locate yourself in your body, allow thoughts of the world outside to recede and bring awareness into your body. Move your awareness around your body taking time to feel the different parts of your body. Allow any thoughts of the world outside to pass.

Tune into the rhythms of the body Like nature, the body has its own cycles and rhythms. Feel the rhythm of the breathing, like the ebb and flow of the tide. Notice the chest rise as the lungs fill with air then fall as you exhale. Our human cycles are also part of the natural cycle.

Pay attention to what you feel Do not attempt to force any changes and be aware of what you feel in different parts of your body. Notice where in your body you feel comfortable, where you notice any tightness or even where you do not feel anything at all. Try not to interpret or analyze what you feel. Just allow the feelings to be.

Stay in the present moment When your thinking is attached to the past or the future, you lose the opportunity to be fully present to the richness of your own experience. Gently bring your attention back again and again to what you are feeling at this very moment. Let thoughts about the past and future go. Stay here in your body now. If thoughts about what you did earlier or what you will do later come into your mind, just let them pass, do not suppress them or give them any further attention. Become aware of the richness of the present moment here in your body.

Suspend your judgment Avoid judging your experience and any thoughts that arise in the meditation. By withholding judgments about your experience, you are more able to fully participate in the present moment. Remember: There are other times for you to reflect on and analyze your experiences, rather than while you are meditating.

A meditation on inner peace Use this meditation at the beginning and the end of the day or whenever you feel tension building and need a refreshing break. Sit in a comfortable position and bring your awareness into your body. Allow the distractions of the world outside to recede into the distance. Be aware of how your body feels and where you are holding any tension. Gently shrug the shoulders and adjust your body for comfort.

Draw your attention inward to the rhythm of your breathing. Notice the rise and fall of your chest with each breathing cycle. Feel the air pass through your nose and fill your lungs. Allow all the breath to be expelled, and with the release of the breath, allow any tension in the chest, shoulders, and neck to be released. Feel the tension falling away with each breath.

Imagine your mind as a screen with thoughts passing across it. Allow your thoughts to pass across the screen without hanging onto them. Feel a detachment from your thoughts, notice them arise in your mind and then dissolve. Feel a stillness in your mind that exists below the level of thoughts. Pay attention to this stillness.

Feel the stillness within you growing. Allow yourself to sink deeper into this feeling. Enjoy the feelings of peace and stillness and allow them to expand to fill your mind and body.

Technique	Awareness and visualization
Time	Spend 15–20 minutes twice a day
Position	Sitting comfortably or lying on your back

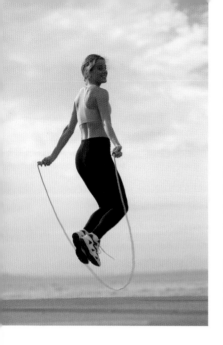

In addition to all the physical benefits, regular exercise can endow you with a more positive mental attitude, and help you combat stress.

Feel this sense of peace and stillness filling each part of your body. Feel your chest filling with this peace. Feel it extend out to your shoulders and neck, down your arms to your hands. Feel it into your abdomen and down your legs.

Enjoy the glow of that peace radiating outward beyond the boundaries of your body. Immerse yourself deeply in this experience of stillness, and imagine feelings of peace emerging within yourself and radiating out to the world.

Exercise

Exercise is one of the best stress relievers, and to get the most benefit you should aim to exercise a minimum of three to four times weekly for 30–60 minutes. A balanced program of exercise includes regular stretching for flexibility of the muscles and joints, strengthening exercises to develop appropriate muscular support, and aerobic activity to stimulate the metabolism and build stamina.

There is good evidence that aerobic exercise (such as brisk walking, cycling, and jogging) has a profound effect on the cardiovascular system and can prevent, and in some cases reverse, cardiovascular disease. In addition to this, aerobic exercise stimulates intestinal activity, helps food waste pass more effectively through the body, boosts the immune system, and enhances mood.

A key to sticking to your exercise regimen is creating one that brings you pleasure. If swimming or jogging is not your choice, then find an alternative activity. Other aerobic activities you might consider are dancing, tennis, and golf. If you cannot find a way of enjoying your exercise, it will be easier to lapse from your regimen. People are usually very committed while the memory of the symptoms are strong, but as the symptoms wane, so can the commitment as other priorities take the place of exercise.

Many of the benefits of aerobic activity can also come from mild fitness practices, such as walking, tai chi, yoga, and qi gong. Whether it is due to health limitations or dislike of more vigorous types of exercise, these gentle methods can bring many benefits, such as improving circulation, enhancing breathing, and focusing and relaxing the mind. You can give real attention to the subtle changes taking place in the body through movement. This quality of attention or mindfulness taps into a deep healing resource. Carefully noticing what is happening in your body is often the first step in bringing about positive change in behaviors. Noticing that your body feels freer and more comfortable after exercise is a great incentive to maintain your regimen.

A breathing exercise (Udiyama) from classical yoga can help stimulate the digestive processes and massage the abdominal organs. The starting posture for this exercise is to stand with your feet shoulder width apart and your toes pointing forward. Slowly bend your knees and trunk forward, placing your hands on your thighs above the knee with your wrists facing outward. Your spine and head should be relaxed and straight. Your shoulders, arms, and hands should also be relaxed as you balance in this position. Make sure you are not leaning too far forward or your buttock muscles will tighten to stop you falling forward. When you are comfortable enough in this position, exhale forcefully emptying your lungs, and push your abdomen out. Keeping your lungs empty, alternately contract then relax your abdominal muscles nine times in rapid succession. The movements should be deep, smooth, and regular. Repeat several times. When done correctly, the contraction of the abdominal muscles will massage the digestive organs. Most yoga teachers do not recommend this during pregnancy or menstruation.

Posture

How you stand and move can also have a profound influence on your digestion. If you are hunched over with rounded shoulder the digestive organs will be crowded and compressed. If the arch in your lower back is too deep, then instead of the pelvic bones acting as a bowl that carries the abdominal contents, they will tend to hang from their ligamentous connections. This is exaggerated if the abdominal muscles lack sufficient tone and are stretched with the abdomen protruding. Disciplines that work with structural alignment (such as osteopathy, yoga, Alexander technique, and Rolfing) can help correct these imbalances and benefit the digestion.

simple
remedies

A balanced diet is essential for health and well-being, and you need to eat a varied diet to ensure that you get the full range of nutrients. These include carbohydrates, proteins, essential fatty acids, vitamins, and minerals. What's more, research over the last 2 decades has revealed that many foods, in particular fruit and vegetables, are rich in additional substances that enhance health.

Make food your medicine

Phytochemicals are changing the way we think about fruit and vegetables. It is clear they offer much more than a source of carbohydrates with a few vitamins and minerals. For example, broccoli contains a substance that may prevent breast cancer. Citrus fruits have substances that make it easier for your body to remove carcinogens, thus decreasing the chance of developing cancer. Grapes contain a phytochemical that appears to protect each cell's DNA from damage. Similarly, a number of herbs and vegetables contain phytochemicals that appear to offer protection against cancer-causing substances (carcinogens). The list is extensive: bok choy, broccoli, brussels sprouts, cabbage, cauliflower, carrots, kale, mustard greens, red beets, peppers, garlic, onions, leeks, and chives are but a few of the herbs and vegetables that appear to have cancer-preventing phytochemicals. There are also a number of foods that have specific properties that can be beneficial for digestive health:

Apples and pears These fruits contain pectin, a soluble fiber, and sorbitol, which is a sweetener with laxative properties. The soluble fiber helps lower cholesterol levels and is useful in preventing gallstones. Eat one or two pieces of these fruits each day.

The soluble fiber in apples and pears will help lower your cholesterol levels. There is some truth in the old adage "an apple a day keeps the doctor away."

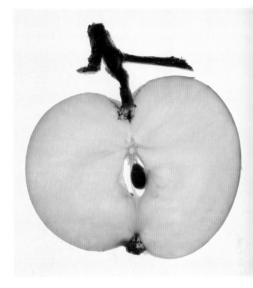

Bananas Bananas are high in potassium and give the body slow-burn energy (unless they are very ripe, in which case they will increase the blood sugar level more quickly). The body loses potassium when you have diarrhea, so bananas can help restore some of this essential mineral. They are also rich in the probiotic FOS (fructooligosaccharides), which provide food for the beneficial bacteria in the gut.

Brassicas These are cruciferous vegetables (such as broccoli, cabbage, brussels sprouts, and cauliflower) and are rich in sulfur (as are onions and garlic). Sulfur is the basis of glutathione, which provides antioxidant protection to the stomach lining.

Carrots This vegetable is an excellent source of beta carotene, which the body uses to heal damaged tissue in the stomach. Carrots are useful for sufferers of peptic ulcers and inflammatory bowel disease.

Cold-water fish Fish provides easily digested protein and many trace nutrients and is low in cholesterol and saturated fats. Cold-water fish (such as salmon, tuna, mackerel, herring, and sardines) are especially rich sources of omega-3 fatty acids, which have a beneficial effect on inflammatory conditions and the cardiovascular system. What's more, including cold-water fish in the diet several times a week may even help the symptoms of inflammatory bowel disease.

Figs and prunes Both these fruits have gentle laxative properties that help the stool move along the colon. They are rich in calcium and potassium. In addition

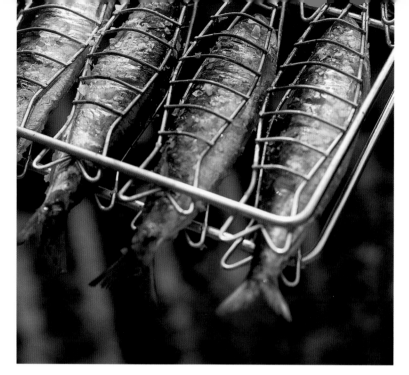

Cold-water fish like these sardines contain omega-3 fatty acids which can alleviate inflammatory conditions. Other cold-water fish include salmon, herring, and mackerel.

prunes contain the antioxidants beta carotene and selenium and dried figs are a good source of iron. Take several pieces each day.

Flaxseed (linseed) Flaxseed produces a fiber gel when swallowed that has a soothing effect on inflammation of the digestive tract. It is very rich in omega-3 fatty acids, which help limit inflammation. In addition, the soluble and insoluble fiber helps with constipation. The whole seed is used, and a typical daily dose is 3 tbs (45 g) per day. It has a nutty flavor and can be used whole or ground, sprinkled directly onto foods. Mixed with an equal amount of boiling water and left to stand for 5 minutes, it resembles a cooked cereal.

Ginger This tasty spice can help relieve nausea and vomiting and has a relaxant effect on the intestine. It has a gentle, stimulatory effect on the flow of bile that can be helpful for indigestion and flatulence. If 2–4 gm of fresh root or 0.25–1.0 gm of powdered root is used each day, it relieves nausea, flatulence, and indigestion. To relieve nausea and vomiting, a small piece of fresh ginger can be chewed or it can be made into a tea by infusing grated ginger in boiling water for a few minutes. If gallstones are present, the use of ginger should be limited to ordinary intake within the diet, rather than taken in therapeutic doses.

Garlic Garlic is an antimicrobial that exerts its effects on a broad spectrum of bacteria, viruses, fungi, and parasites. Its ability to inhibit the effects of *Candida albicans* makes it useful in treating dysbiosis, and its regular use helps prevent parasites getting a foothold in the gut. In addition, garlic brings down raised blood cholesterol and triglyceride levels and can help control raised blood pressure. The active component in garlic, allicin, also has antioxidant properties and can help detoxify various chemicals and heavy metals that can have cancer-causing effects. In populations that consume large quantities of garlic, incidence of stomach cancer is low.

Globe artichoke This vegetable stimulates the function of the liver and the secretion of bile. It is helpful in relieving bloating, loss of appetite, nausea, and abdominal pain associated with gallbladder problems and IBS. It has the additional benefits of lowering blood cholesterol levels and lowering blood sugar levels, making it a useful food for adult-onset diabetes.

Green tea Although derived from the same plant as ordinary black tea, green tea leaves are not left to oxidize. As a result, the cancer-protective polyphenols in green tea are maintained. Both contain caffeine, but green tea has less and some commercial preparations are decaffeinated. The polyphenols in green tea are potent antioxidants and may inhibit the formation of nitrosamines, which can cause stomach and colon cancer.

Papaya Sometimes known as pawpaw, this tropical fruit contains the protein digesting enzymes papain and chymopapain. For indigestion or symptoms of pancreatic insufficiency such as bloating, flatulence, and passing of undigested food in the stool, try including half a small papaya each day in the diet.

Soy foods Some people cannot digest lactose (the sugar in milk) and have signs and symptoms such as diarrhea, flatulence, bloating, and cramping. Soy foods can be a good replacement for dairy products, which have high levels of protein and calcium. Common soy products include soymilk, soy yogurt, tofu (a curd cheese made from soy beans), and tempeh (fermented, partially cooked soy beans).

Whole-grain foods Wheat and rice are two grains that are often processed to remove the fiber, but they provide the greatest nutritional benefit when they are in their unrefined state. As well as supplying carbohydrate, protein, and B vitamins, whole-grain bread and brown rice are rich in insoluble fiber, which is helpful for irritable bowel syndrome (IBS), constipation, hemorrhoids, and gallstones. For some people, insoluble fiber can aggravate a digestive condition such as IBS and should be avoided. Anyone suffering from IBS should ensure they are getting plenty of soluble fiber from dried beans and legumes, fruits, and vegetables.

Yogurt Yogurt that is cultured with beneficial bacteria such as *Lactobacillus acidophillus* can help maintain the healthful friendly flora (providing the yogurt is not then pasteurized, because the intense heat kills the beneficial bacteria). It will also assist in recolonizing the gut following an infection or the administration of antibiotics. Dairy products, such as milk and cheese, are best avoided if the person has an allergy to milk protein or a lactose intolerance. Because yogurt is partially digested by the bacteria, some people with mild intolerances may be able to eat yogurt. If the intolerance is specifically to cows' milk you can try using goats' or ewes' milk products.

Juicing

Vegetables and fruit contain an abundance of important nutrients for the body. In addition to protein, carbohydrate, vitamins, and minerals, juices also contain compounds such as carotenes, chlorophyll, bioflavonoids, and other phytochemicals that support the body's natural reparative processes. When you use a juice extractor, the juice you obtain concentrates the nutrients available to the body. You would have to eat 1 lb (0.5 kg) of carrots to get the nutrients packed into a single glass of carrot juice. The body assimilates the nutrients of fruit and vegetables far more readily when they have been separated from the fiber into a juice. The digestive system has to work hard to break down and digest the nutrients in foods, but juicing gives the body a rest from some of this activity, allowing it to concentrate on healing. The fact that juices are made from fresh raw vegetables and fruit means that valuable nutrients are not destroyed by cooking. Of course the body does need a plentiful supply of fiber, so drinking juice is not a replacement for eating fruit, vegetables, and other fiber-rich foods. Rather it is a complement that provides concentrated and easily absorbed nutrition.

Citrus fruits (grapefruit, oranges, lemons, and limes) provide healthy portions of vitamin C. Carrot juice contains large quantities of the antioxidant beta carotene. Fruit juices are a good source of essential minerals, such as iron, copper, potassium,

Pure fruit and vegetable juices provide an easily digestible source of nutrition.

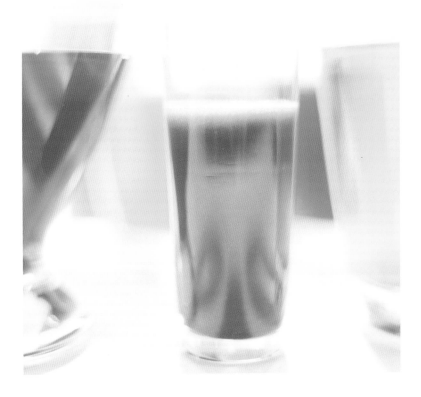

JUICING

Drink your juice slowly, treat it as a food, almost chewing it to savor the flavors. Some good combinations include:

- Carrot, apple, and celery
- Beet, carrot, apple, and parsley
- Papaya and pineapple
- Cabbage (green is best) and apple
- Carrot and ginger

sodium, iodine, and magnesium, which are bound by the plant in a form that is easily assimilated during digestion. Fruits and vegetables are also the source of phytochemicals, which are believed to protect against cancer.

Juicing a variety of fruits and vegetables will give the benefits of the different foods, while avoiding allergic or other reactions that can occur when single foods are eaten excessively. For example, beta carotene from too many carrots can turn the skin orange. There are some specific foods that can have a beneficial effect on digestive disorders. Cabbage juice has been shown to help heal peptic ulcers, and the dose recommended is a cup of juice twice daily for as long as the ulcer persists. Ginger helps digestion and gives relief from nausea and vomiting. It can be added in small quantities to other juices to give a spicy taste.

Guidelines for making juice Wash and peel any fruits and vegetables that you normally would if you were to eat them. For example, remove the peel from oranges but not from apples.

- Small seeds in fruits such as apple or watermelon can be juiced.
- Do not cut fruits and vegetables ahead of time. The fresher the juice, the more nutrients it contains.
- You should consume the juice as soon as possible after making it. The longer it is left (even in the refrigerator), the more nutrients will be lost. If you need to store the juice for a short time, keep it in the refrigerator in a container filled to the top (to reduce contact with air) and add a pinch of vitamin C powder to preserve it.

■ Over a 2-week period, use a wide variety of fruits and vegetables rather than concentrating on just one or two.

Supplements

A balanced diet and lifestyle is the basic requirement for improving your digestive health, but supplements may help restore balance to a disturbed digestive system and treat specific conditions.

Alpha-lipoic acid This antioxidant nutrient assists the liver in its detoxifying function and helps prevent cellular damage to the liver in conditions such as hepatitis. The dosage range is from 100–600 mg daily. This supplement should be used cautiously in diabetics because it can cause hypoglycemia.

Digestive enzymes Enzymes are required to break down the components of food. Amalyse is produced by the pancreas and splits carbohydrates into smaller molecules, lipase breaks down fats, and protease acts on proteins. If the pancreas is producing insufficient amounts of these enzymes, then signs and symptoms such as bloating, indigestion, flatulence, and passing of undigested food in the stool will occur. In the longer-term, nutritional deficiencies will develop. These deficiencies can be supplemented with pancreatic enzymes, which are usually sourced from fresh pig pancreas. There are effective vegetarian sources of enzymes extracted from papaya or pineapple or cultured on molds. These are available in combinations of amalyse, lipase, and protease. It is important to use high-quality supplements that provide sufficient levels of activity. The dosage is based on the level of enzyme activity described as European Pharmacological Units (EPU). To aid fat digestion, take one to two capsules of 10,000 EPU of lipase three times daily before or with meals. To aid protein digestion, take 600 EPU of protease three times daily with meals. And for carbohydrate digestion, take 8,000 EPU of amalyse three times daily with meals.

Bromelain This enzyme is extracted from pineapple stems and has anti-inflammatory effects as well as being a digestive aid. When taken with food, bromelain breaks down protein. The enzyme is useful for pancreatic insufficiency and the gastrointestinal upset that occurs from this. The dosage is 500 mg taken with every meal. As an anti-inflammatory, it can help healing from trauma or surgery. It may also be useful in conditions of the gastrointestinal tract where there is inflammation, such as inflammatory bowel disease. When used as an anti-inflammatory, it should be taken on an empty stomach.

No serious adverse effects have been reported, but mild gastrointestinal symptoms occur occasionally. If this happens, try taking it with a low-protein food, such as fruit. The use of bromelain may maximize the effects of antibiotics and make them more effective.

Papain The protein digesting enzyme extracted from papaya leaf and fruit is known as papain. It may be used like bromelain in cases of pancreatic insufficiency and the gastrointestinal upset that results from this. The dosage is 50,000 EPU.

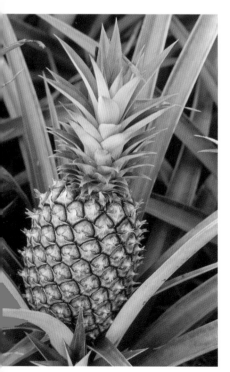

Quercetin The most active bioflavonoid with anti-inflammatory effects is quercetin. It also helps to control the effects of allergies. The dosage is 500 mg taken on an empty stomach.

Betaine hydrochloride Betaine hydrochloride is used when stomach acid levels are low, resulting in belching or burning immediately after meals, a feeling that food sits in the stomach without digesting, and an inability to eat more than small amounts at a time. See the text about hypochloridia on p.43 for information about how to take this supplement.

The enzyme bromelain has anti-inflammatory properties and is extracted from pineapple stems. And the flesh of the pineapple is a delicious ingredient for juicing.

Essential fatty acids Essential fatty acids of the omega-3 variety (from flaxseed oil and fish oils) produce an anti-inflammatory effect by deactivating the pro-inflammatory metabolic cascade from arachidonic acid (found in meat and dairy). The first step in limiting inflammation is to increase your intake of omega-3 fatty acids. This strategy should help any inflammation in the digestive tract— particularly inflammatory bowel conditions such as Crohn's disease or ulcerative colitis.

The two major sources of omega-3 fatty acids are cold-water fish and flaxseed. Most of the research into these remarkable fats is based on fish oils. Flaxseeds provide a vegetarian source, although a series of metabolic steps within the body are required to turn flax oil into eicosapentaenoic acid (EPA), which is the active constituent of fish oils. Fish oils should be obtained from a reliable source as heavy metal pollutants of the sea are concentrated in the fish oils.

The dosage is 3–4 gm of fish oil each day with a standardized EPA content of 1,000 mg or 3–5 gm of flax oil.

Glutamine The amino acid L-glutamine, which is one of the primary fuels used by the intestinal lining cells, can help restore the gastric mucosa. It aids the healing of peptic ulcers (cabbage juice is high in glutamine) and assists in repair of the gastrointestinal lining after damage by infection, drug or radiation therapy, or leaky gut syndrome. Conditions likely to benefit from supplementing with glutamine include peptic ulcers, for which the dose is 500–2,000 mg three times daily on an empty stomach. For IBS, inflammatory bowel disease, or leaky gut syndrome, the dose is 500–2,000 mg three times daily.

Probiotics Lactobacillus acidophilus and bifidobacteria are the two most prominent beneficial bacteria that are normal inhabitants of the gut. Their presence keeps in check a whole range of potentially harmful microorganisms from E. coli, salmonella, and shigella to Candida albicans. In addition to providing a defensive function they also manufacture many of the B vitamins, folic acid, and vitamin A, and they increase the effective absorption of minerals such as calcium, magnesium, iron, and copper. Probiotics also help normalize cholesterol levels and improve peristalsis and bowel transit time. They should be taken after the administration of antibiotics, which kill many of the beneficial bacteria and cause gut disturbances such as diarrhea. The dosage of probiotics for preventive measures should be about 1 billion viable organisms each day. For therapeutic doses this increases to 10 billion viable organisms per day.

Prebiotics These provide the preconditions in which probiotics (see p.109) can survive and proliferate. FOS are natural sugars that are indigestible to humans. FOS act as prebiotics by providing the food on which the beneficial intestinal bacteria, acidophilus and bifidobacteria, live. In addition to increasing the population of these beneficial bacteria, FOS inhibit many of the pathogenic microbes that can cause gut problems such as salmonella, listeria, campylobacter, and shigella. Foods that are particularly rich in FOS include Jerusalem artichokes, onions, garlic, leeks, bananas, and asparagus. FOS are also available in powder form. A dosage between 2–5 gm of the powder per day will help support the population of beneficial bacteria and provide fiber bulk.

Vitamins and minerals

A good quality broad-spectrum multivitamin and mineral formulation is useful health insurance. Even if much of it leaves the body unused, you are providing for deficiencies and extra demand that can occur with illness. It is an unfortunate fact that people's diets do not provide sufficient vitamins and minerals for optimum function.

Certain vitamins and minerals are especially important in digestive health. Deficiencies can occur as a result of digestive diseases affecting the pancreas or small intestine, such as celiac disease or Crohn's disease, as well as severe dysbiosis or allergies.

Vitamin A The recommended dosage is 5,000 IU (international units) per day, except in acute viral infection where dosage can be up to 50,000 IU per day for a maximum of 2 weeks. Vitamin A overdose is a concern because it is included in various preparations for eye, skin, or joint health. Many fish oil formulas contain extra vitamin A. If these are taken together with a multivitamin then the recommended dosages may be exceeded. Women of childbearing age should not take dosages above 5,000 IU per day because large doses have been linked to birth defects. A better choice is to take beta carotene, which is a precursor to vitamin A. It has a similar effect in most conditions, but does not have the potential for toxicity.

Vitamin C The dosage is 500–1,000 mg three times per day. Vitamin C is an antioxidant that neutralizes nitrosamines, which are linked to stomach and colon cancer, and inhibits growth of *H. pylori*. This vitamin is essential for proper healing of damaged tissues, because infection and inflammation rapidly deplete vitamin C in the body.

Vitamin D An intake of 200 IU daily is important for cell growth and regulation of the immune and nervous systems. If there is a problem with fat absorption (as there is in celiac disease, pancreatic disease, or other small bowel disorder), then supplementation is important.

Vitamin E A dose of 400 IU per day enhances tissue healing. Vitamin E is a fat-soluble vitamin like A and D, so it is important to supplement when fat absorption is a problem.

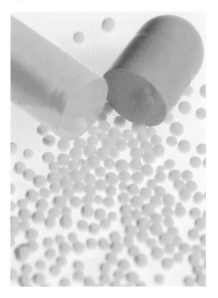

Zinc An intake of 15–30 mg per day is necessary for growth and healing. Zinc is rapidly depleted in the body.

Tests There are various tests that can establish blood and cellular levels of nutrients such as vitamins, minerals,

Vitamin C is one of the most well-known vitamins, recognized primarily for its ability to fight the common cold. But it has many other useful properties.

amino acids, and fatty acids. Although unnecessary for routine use of supplements, tests may be required for diagnostic work by practitioners of nutritional medicine.

Herbal medicine

Many herbs can be helpful in treating digestive disorders, and the following list highlights some of the most important herbs and their uses. Although most herbs are safe when used as indicated, their safety during pregnancy has not been determined. Therefore, anyone who is pregnant or breast-feeding should consult a professional herbalist before using herbs.

Aloe vera Aloe vera is a soothing, healing herb that is helpful in inflammatory conditions such as peptic ulcers or intestinal inflammation. It is best taken as a gel, fresh from an aloe leaf slit lengthways, but commercial preparations, stabilized gel, or juice are available. The dosage is 2 tbs three times daily on an empty stomach or as directed for commercial juices. The latex of aloe, which is sometimes used for constipation, should be avoided during pregnancy because it may cause uterine contractions and miscarriage.

Artichoke Extracts from the leaves of the globe artichoke have been shown to be helpful in the relief of bloating, loss of appetite, nausea, and abdominal pain associated with gallbladder problems and IBS. Take artichoke extract as directed by the manufacturer.

Chamomile Chamomile is used as a tea for its calming effects. It is taken for indigestion caused by the effects of stress. It has mild antispasmodic and anti-inflammatory effects that can help in a range of gastrointestinal conditions, from peptic ulcers to IBS. To prepare chamomile tea, steep 2–3 gm in hot water, and drink three times a day. If it is in tincture form, take 5 ml three times daily. Chamomile tea is safe for pregnant or nursing mothers in small doses, but anyone with a history of miscarriage should avoid it.

Dandelion The bitter components of the dandelion root helps aid digestion. Bitters stimulate the initial phase of digestion by increasing the secretion of salivary and digestive juices, including the release of bile from the liver and gallbladder. If using the dried root, take 2–8 gm as an infusion or decoction (extraction) daily. It can also be taken as a fluidextract, when 4–8 ml is taken daily.

Fennel Fennel seeds are used to relieve gas and bloating, settle the stomach, and improve the appetite. Fennel is safe for children and expectant or breast-feeding mothers. Make an infusion by pouring boiling water over a teaspoon of the crushed seeds and steep for 5 minutes. Take it three times daily. For the nausea of pregnancy, the tea may be sipped throughout the day.

Gentian The plant gentian is used to make a bitter tonic that stimulates the taste buds and increases the flow of saliva and stomach and bile secretions. Gentian may be helpful in cases of poor appetite, indigestion, heartburn, and nausea. Take as a decoction, which is made by boiling $1/2$ tsp shredded root in 1 cup of water for 5 minutes. If a tincture is used, take 1–2 ml three times daily in a little cold water.

Goldenseal Goldenseal is a woodland plant that contains the active alkaloid berberine. It has broad-spectrum antimicrobial effects against bacteria, protozoa, and fungi, including *Staphylococcus*. sp., *Streptococcus*. sp., *E. coli*, *Salmonella*, *Shigella*, *Giardia*, and *Candida albicans*. Goldenseal is extremely useful for travelers' diarrhea or gastroenteritis from food poisoning. Goldenseal is healing to the gut wall and can help in gastric and intestinal inflammations, such as gastritis, enteritis, and peptic ulcers. To make a tea, $1/4$–$1/3$ tsp of powdered root is steeped in a cup of water for 10 minutes. If a tincture is used, take 0.5–1.5 ml. Take the mixture three times daily, and limit its use to 1 month. Acidophillus supplements or yogurt should be taken to restore the proper balance of probiotic flora, especially after long-term use of goldenseal, because the herb can disturb the flora. This herb is not recommended for persons who are pregnant or who have hypertension.

Licorice root Extract of licorice root is very effective in treating peptic ulcers. It does this by stimulating the normal defense mechanisms that prevent ulcer formation, rather than by inhibiting the release of stomach acid as most drugs do. Licorice accelerates the secretion of protective mucus and protects the gastric mucosa. Because some components in licorice can lead to fluid retention and high blood pressure, only the deglycrrhizinated (DGL) extract should be used. To heal peptic ulcers, DGL must mix with saliva. The standard dosage is two to four 400 mg chewable tablets between meals or $1/2$ hour before meals. Once the symptoms have resolved, the course should be continued for 2–3 months to ensure complete healing. The use of licorice is contraindicated for pregnant women.

Peppermint Peppermint can be taken as a tea to promote digestion, settle an upset stomach, and relieve nausea, bloating, and flatulence. The essential oil of peppermint is an antispasmodic and relieves the symptoms of IBS. For this purpose, it must be taken as an enterically coated capsule that will only dissolve when it has passed through the stomach into the intestines. The dosage is 0.2–0.4 ml three times daily, 30 minutes before meals. Peppermint tea is safe for pregnant or nursing mothers in small doses but those with a history of miscarriage should avoid it.

Cammomile and peppermint are just two herbs that can be taken as a tea infusion.

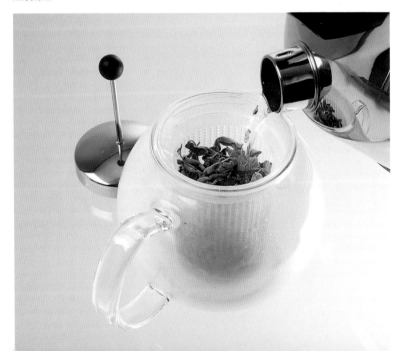

Marshmallow Marshmallow root is soothing to the digestive tract because of its high content of mucilage. It helps in all inflammatory conditions in the mouth and throughout the digestive system. Marshmallow is taken as an infusion, made by steeping 1–2 tsp of the dried root in a cup of cold water overnight. Drink as required through the day to soothe the inflammation. It may also be taken as a tincture; the dosage is 1–4 ml three times daily.

Milk thistle Milk thistle is a Mediterranean plant that contains potent antioxidant flavanoids known as silymarin, which helps regenerate liver cells and inhibit inflammation in the liver. Silymarin neutralizes the toxic effects of various poisons, including alcohol and paracetamol, various industrial and naturally occurring poisons such as carbon tetrachloride, and the death cap mushroom. It is beneficial in most liver conditions including hepatitis, jaundice, and cirrhosis. Silymarin can also help prevent or treat gallstones by increasing the solubility of the bile. A standardized silymarin content of 140 mg per capsule is the best dosage; it should be taken three times daily.

Senna Senna pods are an efficient laxative, useful for the occasional bout of constipation. They should not be taken long-term, because doing so leads to weakening of the muscles in the colon. Senna is available in tablet form from any pharmacy or health food store. The tablets have a standardized sennoside content of 7.5 mg. The dosage is two to four tablets taken at night. The initial dose should start low then gradually be increased if required. Senna is best taken along with a tea made from carminative herbs, such as fennel, ginger, or cardamom. These herbs and spices relax the intestinal muscles, reducing the tendency to intestinal pain and colic.

Slippery elm The bark of slippery elm is soothing and nutritive to inflamed mucous membranes. It can relieve irritation and inflammation of the gut caused by hyperacidity, gastroenteritis, diverticulitis, or IBS. It is made by mixing one part (10–15 gm) of the finely powdered bark with eight parts of water and simmering that gently for 10–15 minutes. Drink $1/2$ cup three times a day. Slippery elm can also be taken as a powder, capsule, or tablet. Tablets contain 2–4 gm and should be taken three times daily for acid indigestion or diarrhea.

Valerian Valerian is a flowering herb that can help reduce effects of anxiety with its gently sedative and antispasmodic effects. It helps relieve cramping and intestinal colic and induces restful sleep, without the hangover effects of many pharmacological sedatives. Valerian may be taken as a tablet of 150–300 mg. The dosage is one tablet three times daily for the relaxant effects on the gut or one dose in the evening 1 hour before bed to help with insomnia. Valerian is very safe, but pregnant or breast-feeding patients should consult a professional herbalist before taking any herbs.

Homeopathy

Homeopathic remedies are very safe and can effectively relieve the symptoms of many digestive conditions. Self-prescribing is not a substitute for proper assessment by a qualified health professional, however. Therefore, if you are unclear about the causes of your symptoms, you should seek the opinion of your health care provider.

Homeopathic remedies are not prescribed exclusively on the basis of named conditions such as peptic ulcer or irritable bowel syndrome. The key to prescribing is to get as close a match as possible between your own symptoms and the specific indications of the remedy. The closer the match, the more effective the remedy will be. Identifying associated symptoms or recognizing what makes the symptoms better or worse may provide the key to the best-matched remedy.

Method and dosages

The remedies should be taken when the mouth is free from food, toothpaste, tobacco, or sweets such as mints. One pill should be dissolved under the tongue.

In acute or recent-onset conditions, the usual potency is 6C for self-prescribing, with the remedy being repeated every $1/2$ to 1 hour up to a maximum of ten doses. As soon as you experience an improvement, the dosage should be reduced to two or three times per day. This may need to be continued for 2 to 3 days. For chronic or long-term problems, 6C may be taken three times daily for up to 14 days. If there is no improvement in the symptoms, you may need to select another remedy.

What to expect

Occasionally, symptoms may temporarily be aggravated as the remedy stimulates the body's healing response. If this occurs, stop taking the remedy. If the condition then begins to improve, you do not need to take the remedy again, but if the improvement stops or slows down, you should start taking it again. If your symptoms continue to get worse, seek the advice of your health professional.

Indications

Listed below are the indications for remedies that relate to digestive health. Remember to look for the description that matches your symptoms as closely as possible.

Abdominal pain

■ Colocynthis for colicky abdominal pains that are ameliorated by pressure or bending over. Vomiting or diarrhea may accompany the pain.

■ Chelidonium for abdominal pain that radiates to the right scapular region. The pain is relieved by eating, and there may be diarrhea with pale stools.

■ Lycopodium for abdominal pain that is worse with deep inhalation. The pain is on the right side and becomes worse between 4 and 8 P.M.

■ Mag Phos for abdominal pain that is better if there is warmth and pressure. Vomiting or diarrhea is milder than in the condition that requires colocynthis.

Constipation

■ *Calcarea carbonica* for constipation without urge for stool. There are general symptoms of weakness and tiredness.

■ *Nux vomica* for constipation with constant, ineffectual urging for stool. There are general symptoms of irritability and quick temper, which are aggravated by overuse of drugs, medications, alcohol, or the strain of mental work.

■ Silica for constipation with the sensation that the stool remains in the rectum after bowel movements. There is a general sluggishness and lack of vitality.

Diarrhea

■ *Argentum nitricum* for anxiety related diarrhea, watery stool with colic, and flatulence, which may alternate with constipation. There are symptoms of fearfulness and insomnia.

- *Arsenicum album* when feeling weak, chilly, anxious, and restless with diarrhea. This is a key remedy for gastrointestinal infections.
- Chamomilla for greenish, frothy stool with severe colicky pains; the stool smells like rotten eggs.
- *Mercurius vivus* for strong urging with offensive, bloody diarrhea.
- *Veratrum album* for diarrhea and vomiting, and collapsed states.

Indigestion

- *Arsenicum album* for burning pain that feels better with warmth. The person will feel anxious, exhausted, and chilly. The symptoms are worse at night.
- *Carbo vegatabilis* for bloating and indigestion that is worse when lying down, and accompanied by flatulence and fatigue. The symptoms are worse in the evenings and out in cold air.
- Lycopodium for heartburn that feels worse with eating, and bloating that is relieved by eructation (belching). Pain or discomfort tends to be right-sided. Symptoms are worse from the late afternoon to early evening (between 4 and 8 P.M.).
- *Nux vomica* for heartburn with cramping and constipation, especially when accompanied by irritability.
- *Arsenicum album* for ulcers with intense burning pains and nausea; take this remedy if you cannot bear the sight or smell of food and you are thirsty.
- Lycopodium for bloating after eating with burning that lasts for hours; take the remedy if you feel hungry soon after eating and awake hungry.

Nausea and vomiting

- Cocculus for nausea and vomiting and the dizziness characteristic of motion sickness, which forces the person to lie down. The sight or smell or even thought of food brings on nausea.
- Ipecac for persistent extreme nausea that is not relieved by vomiting. The nausea is worse when food can be smelled, and there are griping abdominal pains.
- *Nux vomica* for nausea, empty retching, and a sour taste in mouth. Symptoms are a consequence of excess whether caused by food, drink, or mental exertion. The symptoms are worse in the morning, and you may feel irritable and bad tempered.

Over-the-counter medicines

Over-the-counter medicines are available without a prescription at pharmacies and many general stores such as supermarkets and convenience stores. You should check with the pharmacist if you are unsure about using any of the following preparations.

Antacids Antacids are used to relieve abdominal discomfort caused by excess acidity. There are several types of antacids; most are safe for occasional use, but they can cause constipation or diarrhea. If antacids are taken over a long period, they can lead to malabsorption of nutrients (or medicines) and in susceptible individuals they can cause kidney stones. They work by neutralizing the acid and preventing irritation of the sensitive tissues in the upper digestive tract.

■ **Aluminum compounds** (Aludrox, Alu-Cap) are effective in reducing acid, and their action is prolonged. In the short-term, they may cause constipation. Of greater concern is their long-term use at high doses. Aluminium interferes with the absorption of phosphate, and a deficiency of phosphate leads to weakness and bone damage. There is also concern about the link between aluminium and diseases of the nervous system, such as Alzheimer's disease.

■ **Magnesium-containing compounds** (Phillips' Milk of Magnesia) also have a

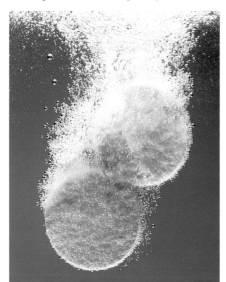

prolonged action and effectively relieve excess acid. In large doses magnesium has a laxative effect, but otherwise it is safe as long as kidney function is normal. If kidney function is impaired, magnesium levels in the blood can build up causing weakness, lethargy, and drowsiness.

Antacids are one of the most commonly used over-the-counter medicines, frequently used to treat overindulgence.

■ **Sodium bicarbonate** is a fast-acting antacid, but its effect soon passes. It reacts with stomach acids to produce gas, which may cause bloating and belching. Sodium bicarbonate is not recommended for people with heart or kidney disease or those on a sodium-restricted diet, but it is safe for occasional excess acidity.

■ **Calcium carbonate** (Tums, Remigel) preparations are fast-acting and effective. A few hours after use, calcium carbonate may produce a rebound effect in which the stomach overcompensates and secretes even more acid. Calcium citrate, which is typically sold as a calcium supplement rather than an antacid, may be a better option. It does not produce the rebound effect, and it is not associated with an increased risk of kidney stones, which are linked to an excess of calcium carbonate.

Many antacid preparations are a combination of the minerals described above with additional substances called alginates or antifoaming agents (Gastrocote, Gaviscon, Rennie Duo). Alginates float on the contents of the stomach to form a protective layer against acid reaching the esophagus and creating heartburn. Antifoaming agents such as dimethicone are included to relieve flatulence (BiSoDol Wind Relief).

Acid-blocking medicines, such as cimetidine (Tagamet) and ranitidine (Zantac), work by blocking the secretion of stomach acid. They are used as prescription medicines to help in the healing of peptic ulcers but have recently been licensed in lower doses as over-the-counter medicines for indigestion, hyperacidity, and heartburn.

Antidiarrheal medicines The first line of treatment for acute diarrhea is preventing depletion of fluids and electrolytes. This is particularly important for children and the elderly, who are more vulnerable to dehydration. Oral rehydration preparations (Diocalm Replenish, Dioralyte) can be used to replace lost fluids and electrolytes. See Signs and Symptoms section for further discussion.

Using antidiarrheal medicines may slow the elimination of microorganisms from the intestine. There are two kinds of medicines that can help with the symptoms. Antimotility medicines (Imodium, Diacalm) decrease the peristaltic muscle contractions and slow the passage of fecal matter. Bulk-forming agents (Fybogel) and adsorbants (Kaolin) absorb water and irritants from the bowel. This leads to larger, firmer stools at less frequent intervals. Antispasmodics are often combined with antimotility medicines (Enterosan, Opozimes) to ease the spasms and pain associated with diarrhea. All antidiarrheals may cause constipation if used in excess.

Laxatives The most common cause of constipation is lack of sufficient fiber and fluids, which was discussed under Signs and Symptoms and in the What to Eat section of Lifestyle Changes. Certain drugs are also constipating, such as opioid analgesics, tricyclic antidepressants and antacids containing aluminium, and ferrous sulphate iron supplements. Laxatives act on the large intestine by increasing the bulk and fluid content of the stool and by stimulating the contraction of the bowel muscles. Bulk-forming agents absorb water from the bowel and increase stool volume. They are relatively slow acting, but they do not interfere with the normal bowel action. Ispagula husks (Fybogel, Isogel) and methylcellulose (Celevac) are commonly used over-the-counter preparations. Flatulence and abdominal discomfort may occur initially. Stimulant laxatives should be for occasional use when bulking agents have failed or a rapid action is required, but they may cause cramping. The most commonly used stimulant laxative is senna. There are various over-the-counter preparations of this (Senokot, Nylax). Lubricant laxatives such as liquid paraffin may be used to soften hard stools that cause pain on passing—for example, when hemorrhoids are present or when there is a blockage of the fecal matter due to impaction.

Medicines for rectal bleeding Treatments for hemorrhoids are for short-term use and are based on soothing agents with astringent properties, such as hamamelis, zinc oxide, bismuth, or Peru balsam (Anusol). Some creams contain a local anesthetic called lidocaine to relieve the pain associated with hemorrhoids (Germoloids).

Prescription medicines

The following medicines cannot be self-prescribed: They can only be supplied by prescription from your medical practitioner. They are strong medicines that must be carefully prescribed to ensure that the risk of adverse effects is minimized.

Anti-ulcer medicines These medicines are used to relieve the symptoms and allow healing of peptic ulcers. A proper diagnosis of this condition should be made by your health care provider. *Helicobacter pylori* is now considered to be the main cause of peptic ulcers, and a full eradication regimen using a double or triple drug combination is the treatment most doctors advocate. The regimen, which lasts 1 to 2 two weeks, is highly effective and should be the first choice for ulcer treatment. The combination therapy is based on an acid-inhibiting drug as well as one or more antibiotics. The type of acid-inhibiting drug currently recommended is known as a proton pump inhibitor, which works by shutting down the acid-producing pumps in the acid-secreting cells lining the stomach.

■ **Proton pump inhibitors** include omeprazole magnesium (Losec), esomeprazole (Nexium), and lansoprazole (Prevacid). Although these drugs are 90 percent effective in 1-week eradication regimens and even more effective for 2-week eradication regimens, adverse reactions may occur. These include stomach pain, nausea and vomiting, diarrhea and constipation, headaches, and hypersensitivity reactions such as rashes and bronchospasm. Gastric acid kills most microorganisms passing through the stomach. Because acid-suppressing drugs lower the level of gastric acidity, there is an increased risk of gastrointestinal infections.

■ **Antibiotics** currently favored for use as part of the eradication regimens are clarithromycin, amoxicillin, and metronidazole. These are effective against *H. pylori*. The most significant adverse effect is hypersensitivity, which can cause rashes and, in rare cases, anaphylactic shock. Because antibiotics disturb the gut ecology various gastrointestinal symptoms may also occur.

■ **Antispasmodics** are prescribed to relieve pain and spasm caused by cramping of the intestinal muscles. They also may help in nonulcer dyspepsia, irritable bowel syndrome, and diverticular disease. Dicyclomine (Merbentyl), alverine (Spasmonol), and mebeverine (Colofac) are commonly prescribed. However, they are sometimes constipating and may cause reactions outside the gastrointestinal tract, such as temporary slowing of the heartbeat (followed by palpitations), dry mouth, flushing of the skin, and dilation of the pupils.

Drugs for inflammatory bowel diseases Medications cannot cure inflammatory bowel disease, but they may be required to manage the symptoms. The primary intention is to reduce the inflammation in the intestine, which is behind most of the symptoms.

Aminosalicylate drugs, such as mesalazine and olsalzine, are effective in limiting the inflammation, but loss of appetite, nausea, vomiting, skin rashes, and headache are common adverse effects. Corticosteroids may be required if the aminosalicylate drugs are ineffective.

Corticosteroids (hydrocortisone, prednisolone, budesonide) effectively reduce inflammation, but they can cause numerous adverse effects including puffy face, excessive facial hair, high blood pressure, osteoporosis, and increased risk of infection. They are only prescribed when the potential benefits outweigh the risks involved. Budesonide, the newest of these drugs, is designed to minimize these systemic (whole body) adverse effects.

Immunosuppressants These drugs act by targeting the immune system, which may be causing or contributing to the inflammation. Azathioprine and mercaptopurine are the most widely used immunosuppressants for inflammatory bowel disease. It can take up to 3 months before these drugs begin to work. Exactly how the drugs work is not clear, but studies have shown they reduce the symptoms. Infliximab (Remicade) is used for severe inflammatory bowel disease that does not respond to corticosteroids or azathioprine.

Drugs for gallstones Gallstones may be present in the gallbladder for many years without causing symptoms. But if they become lodged in the bile duct, they can cause pain, block the flow of bile, and inflame the gallbladder.

Drugs can be used to dissolve smaller stones that are made primarily of cholesterol. The drugs are ineffective if the stones are comprised of other material, such as pigments or calcium. Ursodeoxycholic acid (Urdox, Ursogal) is the main drug used for dissolving gallstones. It works by decreasing the cholesterol content of bile and bile stones by reducing the secretion of cholesterol from the liver. Once the cholesterol level in the bile is reduced, the stones begin to dissolve due to the action of the bile acids. It can take months or years for the stones to dissolve fully. The most common adverse effect of these medicines is diarrhea. For the treatment to be effective, a diet low in cholesterol and high in soluble fiber is required, and this diet must be maintained after the course of medication is completed, because it is common for the stones to recur.

therapies

Western medicine has certainly shown that scientific methods can deal with illnesses previously thought incurable. However, people are increasingly turning to complementary methods for treatment. In recent years, different disciplines have been learning from each other, resulting in a more integrated approach to healing. All therapies covered in this section can help treat digestive ailments; the description of each should help you choose which are the most suitable for you.

Acupuncture and acupressure

Acupuncture and acupressure are drawn from traditional oriental medicine. Their roots go back more than 2,000 years to ancient China. Illness is described in terms of the balance of energy, or qi. This qi, or energy, flow is concentrated through channels in the body called meridians. Meridians are the conduit through which qi reaches all body organs and structures. Symptoms arise when there is either a blockage or deficiency of energy; treatments are then used to unblock or redistribute the energy. In the case of acupuncture, stainless steel needles are inserted into specific points along the meridians. In the case of acupressure, pressure is exerted over specific points and along the meridians. There are various traditions of acupressure, such as shiatsu from Japan and tui na from China.

What to expect An acupuncturist will want to know details of your health history and will ask specific questions about your health and general well-being. The practitioner may want to read your pulse from several points at the wrist and look at your tongue to note its color, coating, and shape. All information from questioning, observation, and palpation is synthesized to build an overall picture of the state of balance in the body. A practitioner of acupressure may ask some of the

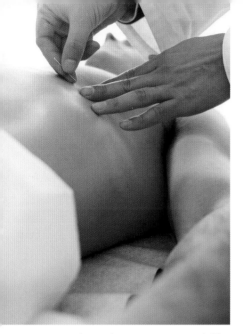

Acupuncture involves the insertion of very fine stainless steel needles into points along the "meridians" to restore qi, or the flow of energy.

same questions but will rely to a greater extent on the findings of palpation.

Acupuncture treatment typically takes place lying down on a treatment couch. The needles, usually 6–10, are inserted into the acupuncture points, and during the insertion process the acupuncturist may twirl the needle gently. You may not feel the needles at all, or there may be a slight twinge or ache as the point is activated. The needles stay in place for 15–30 minutes and, because most treatments are quite relaxing, you may feel sleepy. The needles are then removed and discarded. For certain conditions, the needles are heated with moxibustion. For this technique a compressed ball of dried moxa (the herb mugwort) is held against the needle (never against the skin), creating a heating sensation through the needle. Some acupuncturists are trained in Chinese herbal medicine and may prescribe herbs and exercises (Qi gong) along with the acupuncture treatment.

Acupressure treatments, like most forms of bodywork, take place lying down. Some practitioners use a treatment couch, but most shiatsu practitioners use a mat upon the floor. You probably won't have to undress, but you should wear loose, light, and comfortable clothing. The acupressure massage will be along the meridians of the body. The practitioner identifies imbalanced areas from indications of cold, pain, and stiffness. A typical treatment takes about 1 hour. Although acupressure can be used to relieve specific symptoms, treatments may also be directed toward enhancing a general feeling of well-being.

How many treatments do I need? The number of treatments required depends on the complexity of your illness and your general state of health. Some simple conditions require only one or two treatments to gain effective relief, but chronic problems may need one or two treatments per week for a number of weeks to really improve. You should discuss this with the practitioner before embarking on a course of treatment.

What is acupuncture good for? Acupuncture has been proven to be effective in relieving pain and thus may help with pain caused by digestive conditions. It also has a proven effectiveness in relieving nausea and vomiting caused by surgery, chemotherapy, and pregnancy. Because acupuncture creates quite a powerful relaxation response, it may help in conditions that are aggravated by tension and stress, such as IBS and stomach pain. Acupuncture can be safely combined with other treatments, such as prescription drug or herb therapy, but you should keep your health care practitioner informed.

Herbal medicine

Herbs have been used for their medicinal properties for thousands of years, and each culture has developed unique and sophisticated ways of using plants to treat human ailments. Scientists started extracting and isolating chemicals from plants in the eighteenth century, and mainstream medicine still uses plants as the basis for 25 percent of all medicines prescribed. Examples include digoxin from the foxglove to treat heart problems, opiates from the opium poppy for pain relief, and quinine from the bark of the cinchona tree for the treatment of malaria. Whereas the mainstream approach to medicine has been to prescribe only the isolated active constituent derived from plants, practitioners of herbal or botanical medicine (sometimes known as phytotherapists) have favored the use of the whole plant. Powerful drugs, whether extracted from plants or synthesized in the laboratory, may be effective but not without unwanted adverse effects. Part of the current popularity of herbal medicine has been the belief that these "gentle" medicines do not have the adverse effects that drugs have. Although it is true that most herbs taken in recommended doses are relatively free from adverse effects, some herbs require caution, and plants such as ephedra can be extremely toxic if inappropriate doses are taken.

The use of herbs increases year by year, and in 1998 one-third of Americans used herbs and spent $4 billion dollars on herbal products. Many of these products were self-prescribed. The situation in Europe is similar, but there is one main difference: Along with the self-prescribed herbs, many herbal prescriptions come from health profesionals. A basic training in herbal medicine is part of the standard German medical curriculum. In the United Kingdom there has been a long tradition of training professional herbalists. The National Institute of Medical Herbalists accredits practitioners who complete 3- or 4-year university degrees in herbal medicine. These practitioners have a thorough grounding in all the basic sciences of medicine (including anatomy, physiology, and pathology), but they specialize in using herbal therapeutics. Many acupuncturists have postqualification training in Chinese herbal medicine and their various other systems of herbal medicine, such as ayurveda from India.

What to expect The consultation with a herbalist is a medical one in which details of your health history are explored. The herbalist physically examines you and may order laboratory tests. A typical consultation takes between 30 and 60 minutes. The information derived from this process is assessed to construct an overall picture of how the body systems are functioning. As well as advice about diet and lifestyle, specific herbal prescriptions may be given. The herbalist's approach to devising a prescription is different from a conventional health care provider's. For example, the classic approach to managing an infection is to prescribe antibiotics

Medicinal herbs are often provided in the form of liquid tinctures or extracts.

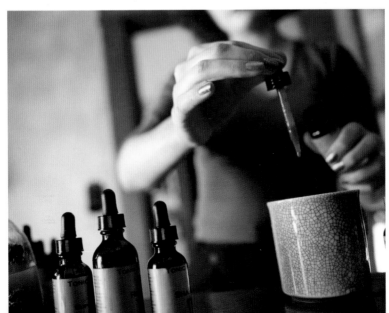

that will kill the disease-causing bacteria. In contrast, the herbalist is likely to give herbs that stimulate the body's own immune response as well as herbs that have an antimicrobial effect. The emphasis of the herbalist is to support the body's own healing response. There are herbs that support the body's immunity, heal damaged tissues, and help the body to process and eliminate toxic substances and to assimilate and digest nutrients more effectively.

Herbalists tend to prescribe combinations of herbs either as a liquid in the form of a tincture or extract or as dried herbs that will be taken as an infusion or decoction at home. Sometimes external preparations are made as creams and ointments. Many over-the-counter herbal preparations come in tablet form. The difficulty with over-the-counter medicines is that there is a great deal of variation in the strength of different preparations and no standard approach to labeling of ingredients. Some suppliers have responded by making preparations with standardized levels of the known active ingredients.

What herbal medicine is good for

Herbal medicine can help a wide range of digestive conditions, from treating indigestion to relieving the pain and discomfort of IBS. Many herbs act directly on the digestive tract rather than through the bloodstream. Herbs such as licorice can help to heal peptic ulcers, and peppermint oil has a direct antispasmodic effect on the muscles in the bowel wall. For minor conditions, self-prescribed herbs can be a gentle way to relieve symptoms but for more serious conditions it is best to consult a professional trained in herbal medicine.

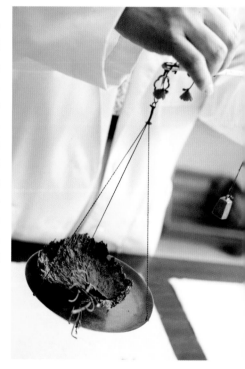

Herbal remedies can be used to treat a wide variety of digestive ailments.

Homeopathy

Homeopathy has been practiced for more than 200 years. It is based on the principle that like cures like. What this means in practice is that symptoms are treated with minute doses of substances that, if given in large doses, would produce similar symptoms to those being treated. The doses of medicine given are extremely small and do not work on pharmacological principles. The homeopathic medicine stimulates the body's own healing response.

This principle of healing was established in the early nineteenth century by German physician Samuel Hahnemann. His discovery of the homeopathic principle came from his own experiments with cinchona (the source of quinine), which was used to treat malaria. He took the cinchona as a healthy person and began to feel feverish, fatigued, anxious, trembling, and extremely thirsty—all of which he recognized as symptoms of malaria. He devised a method of using the medicines more safely by diluting them. The dilutions are made by taking 1 part of the crude substance (typically in a tincture) and mixing it with 9 or 99 parts water. When the dilution is 1 part in 10, the letter X is placed after the number—for example, 6X indicates six stages of serial dilution. When the dilution is is 1 part in 100, the letter C is placed after the number of dilutions. This process reduces the amount of crude material present, but simultaneously seems to increase the remedy's healing power.

Homeopaths have made a systematic study of the characteristics of a whole range of medicines since the time of Hahnemann. Through a careful process of describing the effects of the dilute medicines on healthy people, remedies have been developed that are used to match the symptoms of the individual seeking treatment. The symptoms gathered through this process are not just physical but include mental and emotional states as well as preferences and aversions.

What to expect The homeopathic consultation typically takes $1-1\frac{1}{2}$ hours and explores some of these individual characteristics, in an attempt to find the best match between the symptoms and the prescribed remedy. Sometimes the remedy chosen is a match for the most pressing symptoms, but this may not be completely effective until the homeopath finds a deeper remedy to match your whole symptom picture. Indigestion is a common symptom, and a number of remedies may be used. The characteristics of the individual with indigestion determine the choice of prescription. For example, the remedy ignatia is appropriate for tense, nervous individuals whose indigestion is caused by receiving bad news or a shock, whereas nux vomica is appropriate for forceful, overindulgent individuals who may also be constipated.

What homeopathy is good for Homeopathy may be helpful in a wide range of digestive disorders. It is worth considering for conditions where the mainstream approach is not always effective (such as in allergies, inflammatory bowel disease, and irritable bowel syndrome) or where drug treatments are generally avoided (such as during pregnancy and childhood). For long-term complex problems, homeopathic treatment may take many months, but for simple digestive disorders, the results are quite rapid.

There are a range of remedies that can be used as first aid, and these are available at many pharmacies and health food stores. The usual potency for self-prescribing is 6C or 10X. These numbers describe how dilute the remedies are. The remedies are chosen on the basis of the key symptoms and are taken every 3–4 hours or until the symptoms begin to improve. Because the remedies are so dilute, they are extremely safe, and there is no measurable risk of adverse effects. If the symptoms fail to improve, it may be because the remedy is not the best match for the symptoms. You can try another remedy, but if the symptoms persist, you should seek the advice of a professional homeopath. Refer to pp.117–118 of Simple Remedies for some of the key characteristics of the remedies used in digestive conditions.

Naturopathy

The guiding principles of naturopathy are based on supporting the body's own healing effort. To this end, naturopaths use a broad strategy based on patient education, lifestyle, environmental modification, and a wide range of natural therapeutics, including clinical nutrition, herbal medicine, homeopathy, therapeutic bodywork, and mind-body techniques. Characterized by an approach to healing rather than the use of specific techniques, naturopathy as a specific discipline has existed for about 100 years, although many of the techniques used have a longer history. Naturopaths complete a 4-year medical degree covering the basic medical sciences as well as the application of some of the techniques mentioned here. Some naturopaths are also qualified in other disciplines, such as osteopathy or traditional Chinese medicine and use these as part of their naturopathic approach. It is a whole-person approach rather than a symptomatic approach to treatment. For every illness, the naturopath attempts to evaluate how the individual's effort toward healing can be supported at the biochemical, structural, and psychological levels.

Biochemically the support may come through dietary interventions such as fasting and elimination regimens, vitamin and mineral supplements, and herbal medicine. At the structural level, bodywork techniques may be applied to improve circulation, improve breathing mechanics, and ensure that structural imbalances are not impeding the body's healing effort. Naturopaths have formal training in the psychological influences on illness and may use mind-body techniques to help the individual work with emotional or psychological obstructions to healing. The naturopath is also aware of the importance of environmental influences on health and can help the individual develop strategies to improve either their environment or the body's response to the environment.

THE NATUROPATHIC CONSULTATION

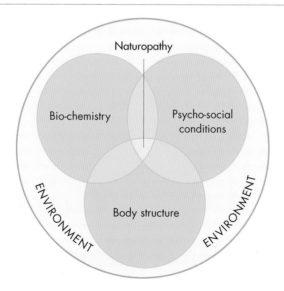

What to expect A naturopathic consultation is much like an extended medical consultation and will include a detailed health history and physical examination. Laboratory testing will be arranged if required.

What naturopathy is good for Because of the breadth of its approach, naturopathy can help in a wide range of health problems, from indigestion to IBS. It can also have an important contribution in more serious digestive illnesses such as inflammatory bowel disease.

Clinical nutrition

Clinical nutrition followed the discovery of the essential role that vitamins, minerals, and other nutrients play in health. The field continues to expand as it has become clearer that nutrients can be used to prevent and treat many more diseases than those classically described as nutritional deficiency diseases. These include scurvy from lack of vitamin C and pellagra from lack of the B vitamin niacin. There is also a growing body of research into the protective effects of antioxidants in cancer and other degenerative diseases.

Clinical nutrition has been adopted into the practice of several disciplines. There are nutritionally oriented medical practitioners and naturopaths who use clinical nutrition as a central part of their practice. Osteopaths and chiropractors as well as other complementary therapists may incorporate aspects of clinical nutrition into their work. There are also dietitians and clinical nutritionists who work exclusively in this field following degree-level training.

What to expect A consultation may take as long as $1\frac{1}{2}$ hours or more to get a full nutritional profile. The nutritionist will want to know exactly what you eat as well as a health history and details of any medications or supplements you may be taking. This fact-finding consultation is followed with specific recommendations on how you can adjust your diet to help with specific health problems. This may include advice not only on what to eat but also on how much and how often. This may be helpful in digestive conditions. As well as dietary advice, nutritional supplements may be recommended for their therapeutic effects. For example, it is well established that fish oils have a protective effect on the cardiovascular system and inhibit inflammation, but you would have to eat cold-water fish on a daily basis to get sufficient fish oils to help in inflammatory conditions. Supplementation with fish oils will ensure your body has sufficient levels of required nutrients to produce the therapeutic effect.

Depending on the nature of the health problem, a follow-up visit after a month would be typical to check on progress and adjust the regimen. Chronic problems need greater input than simple problems of recent onset. A key goal of treatment is to help you establish a healthy lifestyle and good dietary habits.

Mind-body medicine

Mind-body medicine is an approach to healing that recognizes that the mind and body are a fundamental unit and that the mind can be used to help heal the body. Our thoughts and feelings influence the function of the body via the nervous, circulatory, and immune systems. The brain and body are in constant communication through these systems. The brain connects to the body through the nervous system and can affect the behavior of every body system. As well as being the center of the nervous system, the brain also acts as a gland that produces vast numbers of chemicals, which create reactions all around the body. All over the body there are receptors to these brain-made chemicals. The brain also has receptors for chemicals made in different parts of the body. In addition to the activity in the nervous system, there are complex chemical reactions taking place between the brain and the different body tissues that influence body-mind functioning.

There is a large and growing body of research demonstrating how the interactions between the mind, the nervous system, and immune system can affect health and disease. This field is known as psychoneuroimmunology, or PNI. The research from PNI has shown clearly how the mind can be used to heal the body. An example of this work comes from Dr. David Spiegel of the Stanford University School of Medicine. His study in 1989 compared 86 women with late-stage breast cancer. Half the group received the standard care and the other half participated in weekly support groups in addition to the standard care. The women who were part of the support group lived twice as long as those who did not. This dramatic finding highlights the importance that should be given to social and psychological factors as well as physical dimensions of illness.

Over a 30-year period of research, Dr. Herbert Benson and his colleagues have established the efficacy of mind-body techniques in the treatment of stress-related conditions. It is reported that as many as 60–90 percent of visits to physicians are for stress-related complaints. The effects of stress may be experienced at different levels. Your body may tell you before your mind that you are struggling with too much stress. Symptoms include muscle tension, aches and pains, fatigue, and a range of digestive signs and symptoms, such as diarrhea, constipation, and indigestion. Stress is one of the main triggers that aggravate digestive conditions. Stress sensitizes the gastrointestinal tract, not just through the nervous system but also by hormones released within the gastrointestinal tract and other sites in the body.

The field is cross-disciplinary, and practitioners from medicine, nursing, and the range of complementary therapy approaches use mind-body methods. There are also specialist applications in fields such as midwifery to assist in labor and physiotherapy where it is integrated into rehabilitation programs. Practitioners from most disciplines could make use of the techniques of mind-body medicine. The teaching may be of individuals as part of an office visit or as part of a group. Because the field is so wide, no formal qualifications cover all the techniques. A professional qualification in medicine, nursing, or yoga therapy is no guarantee of a practitioner's skill in the methods of mind-body medicine, but it does at least indicate their basic disciplinary expertise.

Various techniques used in mind-body medicine, which for convenience could be loosely classified as falling into four main areas: relaxation techniques, hypnosis, biofeedback, and bodywork.

REDUCING STRESS

A partial list of problems that can be helped by reducing stress include:

- joint pain ■ chronic fatigue syndrome ■ hypertension
- cardiac disorders ■ chronic pain ■ infertility ■ migraine headaches ■ diabetes ■ perimenopause/menopause
- gastrointestinal disorders.

Relaxation techniques This group of techniques includes meditation, autogenic training, progressive muscular relaxation, and massage. Refer to pp. 93–99 for two meditation techniques—visualization and body awareness—that can help you disengage from your usual thought patterns and cultivate a particular awareness of the "here and now." Similar methods are used in autogenic training to induce states of relaxation. Progressive muscular relaxation involves slowly contracting and then releasing each muscle group individually, starting with the muscles in the toes and finishing with those in the head. Massage can be used to induce a relaxation response.

Biofeedback Using electronic monitoring devices, individuals are taught how they can influence body functions that are normally outside their conscious control, such as blood pressure and heart rate. The monitor provides feedback and the individual learns how their thoughts and moods may influence them.

Hypnosis During hypnosis, individuals are guided into an altered state of consciousness where they may become highly receptive to the suggestions that the hypnotherapist makes. This altered state is reached by concentrating on the words or images that the therapist presents, leading to a relaxed but attentive awareness. The next step is suspending critical judgment and allowing the words and images to have their fullest impact. During this stage the unconscious can become highly receptive to the suggestions that the therapist makes—whether they are directed toward bodily functions such as the activity of the gastrointestinal tract or behaviors such as smoking.

Bodywork Touching the body can also touch the mind, and the effects of bodywork can have a profound influence on physical and psychological well-being. Establishing a relaxation response is a common aim for many bodywork disciplines such as massage, but there are some techniques, such as craniosacral work, zero balancing, and hellerwork that specifically use mind-body interactions. There are many dimensions to this kind of work, such as using touch to bypass the rational and conscious mind in a way that helps to reestablish healthier physiological and psychological patterns. Another aspect of bodywork is the way it can bring the conscious mind more fully into the body so that the individual experiences the helpful, and harmful, influences that the mind has on the body, and the body on the mind.

Orthodox medicine

Everyone is familiar with some aspects of orthodox medical care, whether from their general practitioner (GP) or from a specialist. It is, however, worth setting out the distinctive features of the approach and their usefulness in treating digestive conditions. Orthodox, or mainstream, medicine has grown up along with science over the last 150 years. It has used discoveries such as the microscope to peer ever deeper into the body in an attempt to identify the specific causes of disease. The success of this approach comes from analyzing the individual components of disease and looking at the level of the microbe and cell for the causes of disease.

The discovery of disease-causing bacteria and the cellular basis of disease have underpinned some of the phenomenal successes of medicine in fighting what were once devastating and even fatal diseases. Medical education and research has fostered this reductionist approach, and medicine is now divided up into many specialities, because the body of knowledge is too vast for any individual to hold. Most physicians specialize in a particular body system or area. Family physicians or general practitioners are an exception to this rule in that their specialization is to be generalists. They have a good understanding of the processes and management of disease and know how to order tests or refer patients to specialists if greater precision is required in diagnosis, but general practice does not provide precise diagnosis using high-tech equipment.

General practitioners deal with the gray area of human illness, where the spill-over between social and psychological well-being and physical symptoms blur the neat distinctions of disease categories. It is estimated that a precise diagnosis is achievable in high-tech medical centers for about 60 percent of the time, in general practice it is more like 25 percent. Although precision is useful, there is the criticism that in focusing on the disease the person is easily forgotten. Looking at just one area may obscure the whole picture. General practitioners know this and have a pragmatic approach to prescribing. The medicines that general practitioners are trained to use are either for a specific diagnosis, such as antibiotics for an infection, or for a deficiency such as hormones for menopause. Symptom control is also important, using anti-inflammatories, antispasmodics, antacids, or perhaps antidepressants when psychological influences enter the picture.

Your GP will refer you to a specialist such as a gastroenterologist if your condition is not responding to treatment or if a serious disease is thought to be underlying your symptoms. The diagnostic tests that a specialist uses depend on the symptoms, but blood, stool, urine, and endoscopy are important. The section on Tests explains what each is used for. The specialist reports his or her findings and recommendations, and in this way the GP develops an overall understanding of the individual's health problems and is then able to help and guide the individual.

The GP also has a network of individuals or organizations that he or she can refer to, from nurses, dietitians, and counselors for individual consultations to support groups for particular conditions. Increasingly GPs are working with complementary therapy practitioners and in the United Kingdom, it is not unusual to have acupuncturists, osteopaths, and massage therapists working together in the same

Your GP is often the first port of call when you have a digestive complaint.

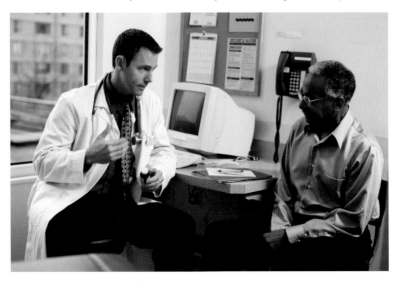

practice. Although the pressure of time may create limits on any single consultation, the role of the GP is intrinsically a holistic one—seeing the links between the different dimensions of health. With increasing collaboration between mainstream and complementary disciplines, the potential for a truly integrated approach becomes tantalizingly close, but having professionals work alongside each other is not the same thing as having them work together in a truly integrated team.

Integrated medicine

The concept of integrated medicine is when the best elements of mainstream, or orthodox, medicine are brought together with the best of the complementary, or alternative, approaches. This is much more than having practitioners of different disciplines working with each other. It requires that they work together with the patient to promote health and deal with causes and symptoms of illness. The idea of working together sounds fairly straightforward, but it is rather like expecting people from different cultures who speak completely different languages to communicate effectively. It takes a lot of effort on the part of individuals to set

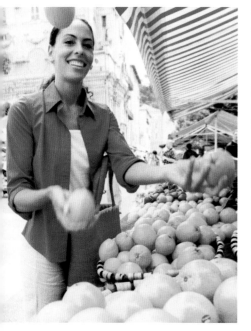

aside their own prejudices and find a common language so they can work together. This is what the people working in integrated medicine attempt to do. They are practitioners from the mainstream who have a broader vision of health care, seeing the body, mind, and spirit as significant contributors to health. They are also complementary practitioners who recognize that every perspective, including their own, has limits and that working together with other professions is the best way to provide patients with the choices they need to move toward health.

Eating a healthy diet is the cornerstone of maintaining good digestive health.

Sometimes drugs or surgery is the only known effective way to manage a disease, and these tools are called on when required. A real strength of the integrated approach is that it is focused not only on disease but also on the resilience of the individual who has the disease. That resilience has a psychological and social component, and the techniques of mind-body medicine are incorporated into an integrated approach. This may be in the form of stress management or relaxation techniques, or guidance toward support groups. Resilience at a physical level depends on maintaining an appropriate level of fitness and exercise, whether in the form of stretching, strengthening, or aerobic activity. Maintaining a healthy immune response is part of physical resilience, and the use of nutrition, herbal medicine, homeopathy, or any other complementary therapy may be integrated into the plan of care. There is also a recognition of the importance of environmental influences and how these can help or undermine our health. In common with naturopathy, integrated medicine looks for the obstructions to healing and helps individuals develop strategies to maximize their healing response. This includes recognizing when environmental toxins are burdening the immune system and need to be removed or avoided, or when the individual's eliminative system is not working effectively and requires support through nutrition, herbs, or other practices.

For medicine to be truly integrated, there has to be real teamwork, because no individual has the expertise of all the disciplines that might contribute to whole-person healing. As well as being experts in their own field, each member of the team needs to have more than a superficial appreciation of how other team members work and how they can best work together for the benefit of the patient.

GPs are well positioned to fill the coordinator role within an integrated practice, but other models of primary care do exist. Individuals may choose to see someone appropriate in the integrated care team—for example, they may see a nurse practitioner for advice, an osteopath because their primary symptom is back pain, or a nutritionist to improve their diet. What is important is that the team works well together and that the patient is central to the decision-making process about the plan of care. There is great potential for integrated medicine, and the few working examples of this are a glimpse into the medicine of the future.

useful organizations

Acupuncture
American Academy of Medical
Acupuncture
5820 Wilshire Blvd., Suite 500
Los Angeles, CA 90036
Telephone: (213) 937-5514
www.medicalacupuncture.org

Aromatherapy
National Association for Holistic
Aromatherapy
4509 Interlake Ave. N., #233
Seattle, WA 98103-6773
Telephone: (206) 547-2164
www.naha.org

Digestive Health
American Gastroenerological
Association (American Digestive Health
Foundation
National Office
7910 Woodmont Ave., Suite 700
Bethesda, MD 20814
Telephone: (301) 654-2055
www.gastro.org

Herbal Medicine
American Herbalists Guild
P.O. Box 1683
Soquel, CA 95073
Telephone: (408) 464-2441
www.americanherbalistsguild.com

Homeopathy
National Center for Homeopathy
801 North Fairfax St., Suite 306
Alexandria, VA 22314
Telephone: (703) 548-7790
www.homeopathic.org

Naturopathy
American Association of Naturopathic
Physicians
P.O. Box 20386
Seattle, WA 98102
Telephone: (206) 323-7610
www.naturopathic.org

Nutrition
American Dietetic Association
216 W. Jackson Blvd.
Chicago, IL 60606–6995
Telephone: (312) 899-0040
www.eatright.org

American Academy of Sports Dieticians
and Nutritionists
P.O. Box 4073
East Dedham, MA 02027
Telephone: (617) 817-0804
www.aasdn.org

General Information
Food and Drug Administration
5600 Fishers Lane
Rockville, MD 20857
Telephone: (888) 463 6332
www.fda.gov

HealthAtoZ.com is a useful website,
giving general information about health
problems
http://www.healthatoz.com

bibliography

The BMA Complete Family Health Encyclopedia. London: Dorling Kindersley, 1999.

Cummings S. & Ullman D. *Everybody's Guide to Homeopathic Medicine.* New York: Jeremy P. Tarcher/Putnam, 1997.

Haas E. *Staying Healthy with Nutrition.* Berkeley, California: Celestial Arts, 1992.

Haas E. *The Staying Healthy Shopper's Guide.* Berkeley, California: Celestial Arts, 1999.

Murray M. *The Healing Power of Herbs.* Roseville, California: Prima Publishing, 1995.

Murray M. & Pizzorno J. *Encyclopaedia of Natural Medicine.* London: Optima, 1995.

Nichols T. & Fass N. *Optimal Digestion: New Strategies for Achieving Digestive Health.* New York: Quill Harper Collins, 2000.

Peters D. & Woodham A. *The Encyclopedia of Complementary Medicine.* London: Dorling Kindersley, 2000.

Werbach M. *Nutritional Influences on Illness.* Tarzana, California: Third Line Press, 1993.

index